The Biggest Little Book About Hope

KATHRYN GOETZKE, MBA

THE BIGGEST LITTLE BOOK ABOUT HOPE

SECOND EDITION

NEW YORK

LONDON • NASHVILLE • MELBOURNE • VANCOUVER

The Biggest Little Book About Hope

Second Edition

Published in New York, New York, by Morgan James Publishing. Morgan James is a trademark of Morgan James, LLC. www.MorganJamesPublishing.com

Proudly distributed by Ingram Publisher Services.

This book is for information only, a personal perspective to share what I know about hope. It should not be used as a substitute for medical advice, counseling, or other health-related services. If you are in crisis in the US, call 800-273-TALK (8255) or text HOME to the Crisis Chat line at 741741. Check out our website at www.ifred.org for additional resources and information.

First Printing: 2020

Morgan James BOGO™

A **FREE** ebook edition is available for you or a friend with the purchase of this print book.

CLEARLY SIGN YOUR NAME ABOVE

Instructions to claim your free ebook edition:
1. Visit MorganJamesBOGO.com
2. Sign your name CLEARLY in the space above
3. Complete the form and submit a photo of this entire page
4. You or your friend can download the ebook to your preferred device

ISBN 9781631958427 paperback
ISBN 9781631958434 ebook
Library of Congress Control Number:
2021951819

Cover Design by:
Arbëresh Dalipi

Interior Design by:
Christopher Kirk
www.GFSstudio.com

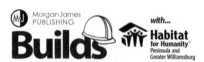

Morgan James is a proud partner of Habitat for Humanity Peninsula and Greater Williamsburg. Partners in building since 2006.

Get involved today! Visit MorganJamesPublishing.com/giving-back

With eternal gratitude to my mom and two brothers, and my nieces and nephew, whose love and support kept me seeing the light even in the darkest of times. To my advisor and mentor, Dr. Myron Belfer, as without your brilliance, compassion, pragmatism, guidance, and wisdom, hope would not be possible for the world. To my second edition editor, Carol Purroy, who encouraged me to put my story where it needed to be. To my fearless writer, Taylor Steed, my assistant, Anna Montances, and my small yet mighty team and iFred board, as without all your love, dedication, faith, and support, this big, bold, bodacious vision of Hope as a Human Right, available free to learn for children around the world, would not have been possible.

This book is to honor my late father, Jon C. Goetzke, and all those we have lost before their time. May all someday know that no matter what life brings, there is always a way from hopelessness to hope.

Love you, Dad.

TABLE OF CONTENTS

FOREWORD

The Biggest Little Book About Hope by Kathryn Goetzke is an intensely personal, easily embraced, story that has universal meaning. Kathryn Goetzke is known globally for her advocacy for suicide prevention and the importance of "hope." This story tells of Ms. Goetzke's journey before and after experiencing her father's suicide. His suicide was a life-changing event as it is for everyone who experiences this tragedy.

Unlike many, Ms. Goetzke has used her experience to forge an incredibly productive life that has aided others. She has shown the way in how to reduce stigma, generate innovative interventions and sustain programs to address suicide prevention. The book is more than a popular "how-to" or confessional. It offers substance to the individual experiencing depression and suicidal thoughts and the professional who wants to know more authoritatively the information about the latest interventions and conceptualizations around suicide. The book is at once both compelling and science-driven.

Drawing on her own experience and working with research collaborators, a sophisticated school curriculum has been developed and evaluated using Healthy Minds concepts. This program has been widely endorsed and supported by international organizations, used along with other potential interventions for all ages, and it gives hope that the future can be positive not only for those at risk but for everyone.

The book provides insight into the latest neurobiological research related to suicide and emotions in a manner that is easily understood. There are valuable references and resource guides for the many areas covered by the book. Interestingly, Ms. Goetzke's acknowledgment section, while meant to thank those who have influenced her life, provides insight into a world dedicated to making people's lives better. It offers a reason for hope.

The Biggest Little Book About Hope is engaging on many levels. As a personal, compelling story, the reader wants to know more about Ms. Goetzke and her life course. As a treatise on suicide prevention, the book provides key information and goes beyond what we now know to suggest what the future might hold. Ms. Goetzke's experience with many modalities of intervention to address the antecedents of suicidal thought and the ways in which the thoughts can be converted into manageable feelings is valuable in the extreme for anyone to know about.

Dr. Myron Belfer, MD, MPA

INTRODUCTION TO HOPE

*All people have is hope. That's what brings the next day
and whatever that day may bring... A hope grounded
in the real world of living, friendship, work, family...*
—Bruce Springsteen

BEFORE HOPE

*Isn't it the moment of most profound doubt that gives birth to
new certainties? Perhaps hopelessness is the very soil
that nourishes human hope; perhaps one could never find
sense in life without first experiencing its absurdity.*
—Vaclav Havel

I was about 24 when my life took an unexpected turn. On a
night while staying at my family farm in Northern Wisconsin that started out like every other night—fun, full of flirting,
with shots and drinks, something happened that triggered the
most intense explosive feeling inside my head, as if a bomb went
off in my brain.

I think it was a disagreement with a guy, and then maybe
with my brother, but I can assure you it was no big deal. The
issue was small, but it struck a very deep chord of pain and alarm
and trauma and isolation. I felt lost and afraid and alone in that
crowded, smoky bar.

"I need out. Now. Of everything. Everywhere," I thought. It was as if I was having a heart attack, yet in my brain. I fumbled for my keys, and ran out into the cold night alone and afraid.

With a deep throbbing in my brain I couldn't explain, I peeled out of the parking lot, internally destroyed, yet unable to reach out to anyone because I could not think and did not know what was happening. All I knew was I needed the pain to end, and felt help-less to do anything about it.

I left the bar, and headed toward home in Minnesota, barely able to see in the pitch black of night, heading on a 2½ hour drive through backcountry winding roads in Northern Wisconsin. I could barely see, my hands clenched on the steering wheel.

The world was closing in, suffocating me with a desperate need to escape. After a few miles of driving, I realized I could not make it in my inebriated and confused state of mind. So I pulled into the ditch, and turned around to get myself back to our farm where I was staying at the time.

Stumbling into the house, I moved slowly despite the internal panic pulsing a million miles an hour through my body. Debilitat-ing, compulsive, loud thoughts raced through my mind. "How can I make this end? I need out. Stop this. Now."

I sought the brown cedar bathroom cupboards, grabbing whatever I could. This amounted to two club-sized bottles of sleeping pills and a bunch of random whatever-else-I-could-find. With my forehead leaning on the cold porcelain sink, I alter-nated between swallowing handfuls of pills and lapping bitter well water out of my cupped hands. I finished off the two giant bottles, and a bunch of other random packages of who-knows-what, hoping it would bring me peace. I then threw myself on the bed, ready to escape my pain once and for all.

I had no thoughts of others, of what I was doing, or how it might impact anything else in my life: My dream marketing and branding job at American Express that I loved, the Master's Degree in Business which I'd begun working on to create social impact products, the friends and family who had stayed with me through thick and thin. These joys were nowhere to be found in these dark, lonely, terrifying moments.

After collapsing on my bed, I drifted off into the abyss.

The next thing I knew, I was floating above that 4-poster canopy bed, looking down with complete love and empathy at a broken, sad, and scared little girl—the girl who had lost her father too soon, the girl who tried and failed to save him, the girl now so unsure of her path in this world, the girl left without her father's guidance.

As I watched from above, I felt no pity, only love. I lifted her up with gentle arms and guided her down a steep staircase that had no rails, in the dark of night, and held back her hair as she released years of despair into the toilet. I felt her gasping for air, and told her it would be all right. When she was done, when she had released it all, I then gently guided her back up those stairs, tucked her under the covers as her dad used to do, and sent her off to sleep, ensuring that she would awaken the next day.

And awaken I did, late in the afternoon. I got out of bed and quietly left the farm, avoiding contact with my brother, driving in shocked silence back to Minnesota. It would be 10 years before I ever told another soul.

See, it was only maybe five years before that I had called home, a freshman at college, to talk to my dad. That day I will never forget, as that day forever changed the trajectory of my life. For when I called, it wasn't my dad's voice that answered the phone, it was another man I didn't know.

He asked who I was, and then I heard him ask for my mom. My mom's voice was shaking on the line, and she told me my dad had died. That he had taken his own life.

I remember the phone bouncing out of my hands, on the cold, hard floor. I remember falling to my knees, my screams reverberating throughout my dorm at Slater Hall in Iowa City, IA. At that very moment, I felt my life was over, in one call, yet knew I somehow would carry on. Somehow, some way.

Never in a million years did I think I would make that same choice, several years later. Never did I think I would do what my dad had done to me to others in my life. I never thought I would make another person feel that pain, that piercing, stabbing pain that ripped my heart out of my chest that day I lost my dad. And then, there I was five years later, having made that same choice and having almost done that to everyone I loved with all my heart.

Only to be saved by an Angel.

It took me another 10 years to even tell another soul that story. To finally come to terms with what happened, and realize that if I wanted to stay alive I needed to start unraveling the puzzle of my mental health, suicide, and the human soul.

I was unwilling to become another statistic. And every doctor, article, and study that I read stated that with my multiple adverse childhood experiences (ACEs), addictive tendencies, genetic predisposition, previous attempt, and multiple major life events, my probability of dying by suicide was very high.

I became committed, on the day I started my nonprofit, to beating the odds and saving my own life. I got sober, started my nonprofit, and got to work on understanding what makes the human soul want to stay alive.

And that is how I found hope.

REBRANDING DEPRESSION

I made my decision to tell my story as I was sitting in Naples, FL on Thanksgiving vacation, just off the phone with my bank. They had frozen my assets for an unpaid tax liability that I thought I had resolved—someone had filed taxes in my name the previous year.

Now, most people might say, "I will have to give them a call to clear that up." That makes sense. It is rational. It is the next logical step.

Unfortunately, that's not how my brain works, especially at that moment. I've worked so hard to get my finances in a good place and have dealt with one issue after another these last few years. This just feels like *one more thing*. I go from hope to hopelessness in .000001 seconds flat.

Instead of thinking I should make the call, my mind jumps into fight or flight mode. And do you know what the first thought is that goes through it? I want to hop on a plane, go home and die. Literally.

It's like a pilot who takes over the plane, gets on the loud-speaker, and says: "This is it. You can't do this anymore." Yet it is my voice. It is me saying it.

I am overwhelmed as a million thoughts snowball into, "I am not meant to be on this planet." It is an immediate and over-whelming switch to panic and despair. Hopelessness at its finest, and almost a reflex in my brain.

The irony is palpable: I'm on an extended break to stay with my mom and write my book on hope, yet here I sit in this state of hopelessness and wanting to die because of one little issue that feels like the world.

Thankfully, I absolutely love irony, and have enough tools in my toolbelt to know 'this is what my brain does.' And the good news is that it only lasts for a few intense minutes, until my *Superhero for Hope* arrives, giving me the tools I need to carry on.

I can't say for sure why this hopelessness happens, but I now have more control than ever, thanks to what I've learned through my exploration of hope. Even with an abundance of risk factors for suicide, including a family history of suicide (genetics, losing my father and aunt, and possibly their father), my own previous suicide attempt, a history of depression / anxiety / addictions / PTSD / ADHD, and multiple ACES, along with challenging major life events and childhood trauma, I am hopeful. I practice and use my tools every day.

I know for sure that if I let my mind run loose, it would, without a doubt, self-destruct. Yet, I have found, through research and practice, that I have more control than I give myself credit for, which in psychology we call self-efficacy. And by the grace of a force much bigger than myself, I found hope. And that has made all the difference.

Let me be clear. The hope I found isn't the "Oh, have a little hope" kind. Besides, that isn't even really hope.

It is the real, actionable, measurable, practical, implementable version of hope I apply to all aspects of my life, from finances to relationships, to work, to eating, to anything, I use my Hopeful Mindset to achieve results. When I don't, I suffer the consequences—but I can always find my way back. Hope is pretty incredible in that way.

My dad's last note to me was for Valentine's Day. In it, he stated, *"I __hope__ and pray you will never experience the pain and __unhappiness__, the deep regret, that I feel all the time."* As I reread that sentence now, it shocks me how it really has become the purpose of my life.

The reality is that I have, at times, and often still do, feel a lot of pain. And even, to my own shock, had an attempt at suicide. However, I refuse to follow in my father's footsteps, and seek so passionately to understand how suicide happens, to prevent it for myself and others.

I saw, so clearly, that his pain was temporary, as has been my own. It always, always, always passes. Yet, we lose too many to suicide every day.

As a result of these experiences and observations, I have made it my own life's mission to figure out what will keep me alive and what ultimately allows me to experience happiness. I truly want to be here. I really want to enjoy life. I want to *experience* life. I want to *feel* life. The good and the bad.

From the day I was born, it was very, very hard for me to sit in any emotional pain—mine or that of others. I always felt like it might kill me, or that I needed to fix it. Immediately.

Ironically, it was my attempt to escape from that pain that almost killed me. I learned over time that I could sit in pain, my own and others, and survive. So, I wanted to learn then not just how to survive, but also how to be present, engaged, and happy.

The insatiable desire led me to create my company, The Mood Factory, as I wanted to learn how to not just be here, but how to enjoy being here. What impacts how we feel? How can we actually enjoy being in the present moment?

The Mood Factory is based on sensory engagement. There is a recent Harvard study that says most people are removed from the present moment an average of 50% of the time, and research suggests this is one of the most significant barriers to happiness. Regardless of what we are thinking about, we are less happy (even if it is a positive memory) than if we are when we are present. Yet those of us that have experienced trauma check out of the present all the time.

I also found one of the easiest ways to be present is through the senses, and the more senses we engage to achieve a desired result, the more powerful it is. I found that not only can we experience presence, but we can also make it enjoyable in what we choose to see, hear, smell, taste, and touch. What a concept.

At the same time as launching my company, I wanted to donate to a nonprofit for mental health for the dual purposes of working to end stigma and raising money to research the cause. I found the branding around mental health incredibly negative and depressing, focusing on the symptoms of depression as opposed to the fact that depression is very treatable. So after many dead ends in creating a nonprofit with potential partners, and my inability to convince them of the need for a mental health rebrand, I ended up creating my own, iFred, the International Foundation for Research and Education on Depression.

I named it after my brother, Fred, because he helped me through my own depressive symptoms at a young age. I then created the acronym, iFred—The International Foundation for Research and Education on Depression. In the first 10 years, my nonprofit was used to present the rebranding of mental health to other organizations and individuals, and teach other nonprofits the 'why and how' so we stopped doing harm to mental health. Rebranding included celebrity engagement, speaking on the biology of the brain (It isn't a choice, though behavior does matter. More on that later.), using universal symbolism (we use the sunflower as the symbol for hope), implementing Cause Marketing programs to increase awareness with consumers (now called social impact), using positive imagery, working on prevention, and teaching other mental health nonprofits the importance of branding.

My first lesson on rebranding, when I managed a project to rebrand IDS mutual funds to American Express, served me well. It taught me how important branding is for the overall success of a product. For example, when I changed the name of our mutual funds from IDS to American Express, we raised a ton of money. It had nothing at all to do with fund performance, as the mutual fund ROI didn't change, it had to do with the trusted name and brand.

When I initially googled 'depression,' I was shocked by what I found. Still, to this day, the images are pretty sad. However, when you do the same for "cancer," the images are much more uplifting and hopeful. Where would you invest your funds? What looks treatable? Do you think you can have an impact?

Further, can you identify with those images? I know that is not what my dad looked like, and not what I looked like, when I had depression. I wasn't holed up in a corner on the ground alone; I was in society, doing my best to hide my pain and suffering. I realized that rebranding mental health with imagery more reflective of those with depression and anxiety was important for both the funds and people's willingness to identify with anxiety and depression, the first step to getting people into treatment.

My initial product line, Mood-lites, from my company, The Mood Factory, got some real success. I did celebrity gift suites, was in major publications, and got in a number of retailers, doing campaigns like 'pink porches' for breast cancer, creating projects that spoke of co-morbidity of depression and other diseases, and spoke anywhere I could about mental health.

I ultimately got Mood-lites in Lowe's Home Improvement stores. I redid the colored lighting category, we doubled sales on a stock keeping unit (SKU) x SKU basis, while simultaneously raising over one million dollars for charities, part of which went to iFred. We proved that consumers were willing to pay more for a product to support a cause while lighting porches blue for autism, and pink for breast cancer, also increasing in-town activism. It was good for all parties involved.

It was social impact before it was a thing. Cause Marketing was typically something big brands did, not start-ups. Yet I lived in the big brand world, having launched marketing campaigns in Alternate Channels for Unilever, Johnson & Johnson, Gillette, and more. And having been trained in business school to take risks, and working for big brands already, I really didn't know any better, nor did I think failure was an option.

It was ironic how I also didn't fully consider the impact of talking about 'mental health' on a brand, as the negative branding associated with mental health impacted my ability to get in retailers. 'What is iFred', they would say? I even had one retail channel tell me I couldn't talk about my social impact model on live TV, even though they allowed others to do so with other diseases. This was in 2008, and it really made me realize just how far we had to go to take brain health to everyday conversations.

Thankfully, we got the brand in retail and got some initial funding, where I could finally put money into what I cared about and what others at the time were unwilling to fund; prevention.

FINDING HOPE

The new funding for iFred meant we could take on an innovative issue for mental health. I really wanted to get to the bottom of suicide. There was a lot of focus on suicide prevention at times of crisis, like restricting access to means and providing hotlines, yet I wanted to explore how we might prevent suicide before it came to a crisis situation. Thankfully, the iFred Board of Directors agreed.

See, I could ruminate myself into a depressive episode, so I wanted to learn all I could about what caused depression in the first place and explore whether it could be prevented. How do I get myself into that state? Is it a healthy human experience, or do I cause myself extra stress?

And I really wanted to know, why do humans take their lives? Why did I try, even though I knew it was an imperfect solution and caused so many others pain? What was really happening in my mind? Why did my dad make that choice, when so many others around him don't?

I also knew that if I really wanted to prevent what many experts say is bound to be my own fate—dying by suicide—I needed to get extra-serious about figuring out how to prevent it. So, I became my primary case study. And I started doing intensive research.

I was encouraged to learn that the only single consistent pre-dictor of suicide was hopelessness, the primary symptom of depression and anxiety. That gave me extreme focus and, with ADHD, my superpower is hyper-focus.

It was even more promising to come across research that suggested hope was something people were studying, and measuring. And it predicted all kinds of positive life outcomes, and was a known protective factor for anxiety and depression. Since there was plenty of research around what raised people higher on the hope scales, we just needed to create lessons to teach it.

For the life of me, I couldn't understand why someone hadn't already operationalized hope. I think this is where my logic course at my local junior college came in handy after I lost my dad. It was one of my favorite courses in college, and has continued to serve me well.

If hopelessness is a key predictor of suicide, let's teach everyone what it is. And what hope is, and how to get from hopelessness to hope. I really could not understand why someone hadn't already done it, as it seemed like the most logical thing in the world.

I had the good fortune of finding an incredible advisory board that was willing to share their expertise: teachers, therapists, youth, psychiatrists, researchers, happiness experts, friends, nutritionists, and more. I hired a tiny team, and we poured all of our funding into using all the available research to create the first-ever free global program to teach hope.

We aimed high, wanting to create a curriculum that could be used around the world for free and be easily adaptable in different cultures, all of it self-led, so that if we ran out of money, the program would live on. I used all my dad taught me about business to make it so, and I'm so grateful to say it does. While there is much I want to improve, we have all that we know open-sourced, online, and available to all. To those who use it, we just ask for attribution of our name and materials, so we can help spread the message.

We initially named the program Schools for Hope (renamed Hopeful Minds), and piloted it in Chicago as a 10-lesson program. We created our own survey and tested comprehension, solving each challenge along the way—things I would come to know as critical to maintaining a hopeful mindset. It's funny, as with any research project, you test the hypothesis (hope is teachable), then get as much data as you can, and improve.

We wanted more psychological research on anxiety, depression, and hope in youth, so we kept a positive attitude—if it was meant to be, it would be. And, thankfully, one day an energetic and inspiring change-maker by the name of Marie Dunne, out of Northern Ireland, asked the same question. By the grace of Google, she asked, "Is hope teachable?" in that little search engine bar and found our site. It was then that our research journey began.

Dr. Karen Kirby, of Ulster University, took charge and agreed to do the initial research, out of the goodness of her heart and the kindness of her soul. She is a kindred spirit, a soul sister who has made this path a grand adventure. Her research has been crucial to the journey and has continued to inform the resources we create.

We've published in journals, and were able to show that as we increased hope in young kids, symptoms of anxiety and depression decreased. We moved from 10 lessons to 12 lessons, based on focus groups with kids. The BBC did a documentary, "Teens on the Edge," showcasing the need for the program and its impact on students, teachers, and parents.

When we received additional funding in 2019, we created both the Hopeful Minds Overview, a 3-lesson introductory curriculum for 2nd-grade students, as well as the Hopeful Minds Deep Dive, an updated 16-lesson curriculum for 5th-grade students. We added a Parent's Guide, so parents could start using hope language at home. We now offer it free for anyone around the world to use, at hopefulminds.org.

We also started two new programs: Hopeful Cities and Hopeful Mindsets. Hopeful Cities is a playbook that provides free resources for cities to activate hope city-wide. The Hopeful Mindsets Training Program is an online platform that provides the "how-to" of hope to different target populations. While both of these programs are still being developed, I am excited to see them reach people around the world as they continue to grow.

Along the way, thanks to the introduction by Dr. Pamela Collins, I met the brilliant, kind, and inspiring Dr. Myron Belfer, a Harvard Catalyst, who is a living hope miracle. He is a world-renowned Child Psychiatrist and used what he has learned from the late Nobel Prize-winning Dr. Joseph E. Murray, who used 'future orientation' with patients, to inspire discussions around hope with academia. Dr. Belfer has given credibility to the construct of hope that I never could have done on my own and gently keeps me on track and moving forward. He has become like a father to me, and words cannot express my gratitude. He has helped move hope along.

Dr. Belfer brought me Kristy Stark, a kindred spirit who goes out of her way to make hope happen. These two collectively shared what they knew about hope and allowed me to join them in presenting on the subject of hope, in the belief that we are stronger together. We have presented at Harvard and several conferences. (Some talks are available at www.hopefulminds.org). Kristy has been a real champion and advocate for hope. She is also brilliant and hilarious, which makes the journey even better.

Dr. Kirby led the charge in Northern Ireland, and published our first paper on our program, looking at pre- and post-intervention (our program) results. The analysis showed a reduction of anxiety and depression, and an increase in emotional regulation with youth.

Dr. Kirby published a second study in 2021, which found that teaching hope to youth improved their well-being, as well as protective factors related to anxiety, depression, resilience, positive emotion, reduced negative emotion, emotional control, stoicism, social support seeking, and self-care. While our program is far from perfect, it is bringing us closer to my global dream of making hope free and available to all—hope as a human right.

It is SO EXCITING, as we are learning that yes, indeed, hope is teachable.

What has become increasingly clear on my journey to hope is the need to get serious about it. As I dig into the research on hopelessness—violence, aggression, addiction, and loneliness—I find that all have their roots in hopelessness. We can't get people to connect if they do not have hope. So, by teaching these skills of hope, especially before the age of 10, we can have a massive positive impact on humanity way beyond mental health.

While Hopeful Minds started out as a tool for preventing suicide (namely, my own), it has turned into a mission to change how we look at so many of life's challenges: homelessness, global warming, poverty, abuse, addiction, and so much more. If we have a goal of solving these issues, we can't do it unless we use a hope framework: Positive Mindset and Inspired Action. It is my intention to share with you some of the insights we have learned along the way.

This book is science-informed, yet I have tried to write it so it's easily understood. I've attended the Mental Health Gap Action Programme (MhGAP) forum for several years at the World Health Organization, learning from leading experts in mental health. I've immersed myself in conferences in the global community. This book is based on an extensive look at hope and mental health globally, blended with my own 'Ph.D. in lived experience', and a need to simply share what we know now to help as many as possible.

My greatest wish for this book is not to *give* you hope. Rather, it is to teach you how to create hope within yourself and apply it to your own life. It is to empower you with tools, so that you may spread hope and empower a child, a neighbor, a friend, a colleague, or anyone else who may need hope in their life. It is to arm you with knowledge, so that you may incorporate hope in all that you do in this world.

Thank you for joining me on this journey to hope.

WHAT IS HOPE?

Hope is the thing with feathers that perches in the soul—and sings the tunes without the words—and never stops at all.

—Emily Dickinson

As I mentioned, hope is not some 'soft, pink, fluffy' concept or soft skill. That is something popular media, and our own misunderstanding, have projected. The word itself needs a rebrand, so try not to let the first thing that pops into your mind influence you.

Hope is small but mighty. I would even argue that hope is more powerful than grit and resilience combined, because, without hope, grit and resilience do you no good. Hope is a building block for everything in life, and without it, we fail to evolve and move humanity forward.

There are many ways to define hope; in simplistic terms, I define it as a vision for something in the future that contains both *feeling* and *action*. To take it a step further, it is a *positive* feel-

ing and *inspired* **action.** If you take nothing else away from this book—know that to hope for anything, you must create positive feelings *and* apply inspired action to move forward.

I came up with this definition based on what it is not. Namely, hopelessness. Hopelessness, as defined by Abramson, is emotional (despair) and motivational (helplessness). So, in very, very simple terms, we must consider feelings and actions when we look at hope and hopelessness.

This is how my work in global mental health has really evolved. I think the field of mental health does a great job of looking at despair, and figuring out how to get support. And I believe scientists that study hope do a lot of work on the motivational aspect (goal-setting). Yet the two are not often combined, and I think both are equally critical, and must both be integrated in the work on hope.

To delve deeper into my own definition, I see hope as a vision, using positive emotion, plus inspired action, as it truly encapsulates the key elements of these words:

- **Vision:** the ability to think about or plan the future with imagination or wisdom
- **Using:** as a means to
- **Positive:** a good, affirmative, or constructive quality or attribute
- **Emotion:** a natural instinctive state of mind deriving from one's circumstances, mood, or relationships with others
- **Plus:** with the addition of
- **Inspired:** of extraordinary quality, as if arising from some external creative impulse

- **Action:** the fact or process of doing something, typically to achieve an aim

The Webster dictionary calls hope "*a feeling of expectation and desire for a certain thing to happen*," yet I believe this is lacking in action, which is necessary, and positive. Feeling without action is often what hope is referred to in society, yet it's not what is measured when we use "hope scales." Feeling, with the wrong action (i.e. uninspired and/or from an angry state) also leads to negative outcomes, and again, not what we measure as it relates to hope.

Dr. Anthony Scioli, a world-renowned hope expert, explains that hope is part of a person's character or personality. You are not born with hope. It must be developed, like a set of muscles. Dr. Scioli defines four kinds of hope: Attachment, Mastery, Survival, and Spiritual. Each type of hope, just like each muscle, has a special purpose:

1. *Attachment hope* is used to build and maintain trusting relationships, have a sense of connection to others, and have strong survival skills.
2. *Mastery hope* is used to become strong and successful, supported in your efforts, and inspired by good role models.
3. *Survival hope* is used to stay calm and find ways out of trouble or difficult situations. It allows you to manage your fears.
4. *Spiritual hope* is used to feel close to nature and all human beings, as well as to draw extra strength and protection.

You'll see much of this sprinkled in our work. In terms of 'spiritual,' we focus more on connection, sacredness, wonder, and awe.

We understand the importance of spirituality and inclusivity, and I personally believe spirituality is key to my own ability to hope. Yet it is also true some may have a negative association with spirituality or organized religion, and I believe hope is an equal opportunity for all and not exclusionary. We have found, as discussed later, that this sense of something greater than ourselves is critical to hope.

The late Dr. Shane Lopez, another leader in hope, says that hope is the feeling you have when you have a goal, are excited about achieving that goal, and then you figure out how you achieve it. He wrote a number of books about hope and studied under C.R. Snyder, another important hope researcher who has added so much to the field.

Lopez's work focused primarily on goals, pathways, and agency. The one thing we've added to our work, as it relates to Dr. Lopez, is more focus on feeling good, and now wonder and awe. We believe these are also keys to maintaining, sustaining, and growing hope.

Dr. Lopez and Dr. Scioli were both kind enough to speak with me as I started on my journey, and they supported my vision of teaching hope globally. I'm grateful to all they added to this program and our knowledge, and for their encouragement. Sadly, as we've been on this journey, we lost Dr. Shane Lopez. This book pays special tribute to him and all he contributed to the field. We are forever grateful to his vision for hope. May it live on through this work and the youth who carry it forward.

When looking at hope, it is also important to look at what it isn't: Hopelessness. Hopelessness has been defined as a negative expectation toward oneself and the future (Kazdin, Rodgers, & Colbus, 1986). It includes both a lack of motivation (helplessness) and negative emotion (sadness and self-loathing) (Abramson, et al., 1989). This again affirms the need to teach hope from both an action (hope as a verb) and positive emotion (hope as a noun-happiness, confidence, and self-love) framework.

While the long definitions are helpful in understanding hope more deeply, most simply, hope is about having a positive expectation for the future and the ability to get there in a way that feels good. If there is one thing you remember about this book, remember this: hope is about both a *positive feeling* and *inspired action*.

So, if we want to teach hope, we've got to teach these two things: how to have positive feelings, and how to take inspired actions. Successfully. And, of course, what to do if you can't do either.

The 'feeling' part of it cannot be underestimated—it is where I believe a lot of us get led astray. For example, if we hope to get straight A's, it is commendable. However, if we treat other people poorly along the way to getting those straight A's, we ruin relationships and isolate ourselves.

If we work so hard on school that we miss out on life and fun experiences, reaching our goal doesn't meet the positive feeling part of hope where we need to enjoy life along the way. As many famous athletes will tell you, it isn't reaching the goal that feels the best, it is how we treat ourselves and others as we move towards that goal. Once we get there, on to the next.

We may also run into challenges when we say things like "I hope to win the lottery," since the likelihood of that happening is rather slim. Though we may 'hope' for it, the ability to actually win the lottery is very unlikely. Worse, if we have pinned our hopes on winning the lottery for retirement, we may receive a shocking awakening when it doesn't happen. We must take realistic and inspired action to anything for which we hope.

What I have also found about hope is that we lose out when we attach hope to a specific outcome. The theory on nonattachment in Buddhism enhanced this understanding for me, as I used to experience a lot of pain when I attached myself to specific outcomes. When we do this and are devastated if we don't meet that specific outcome, that devastation leads down a rabbit hole of hopelessness.

Take a relationship, for example. I might *hope for* a romantic relationship with someone. Once that hope is met with a relationship of my own, I may become highly attached to my significant other—let's call him Hermes—and our relationship. Then, one day, Hermes decides he doesn't like me. I feel hopeless and that my life is over, because I don't have Hermes. I am attached to him.

Yet the reality is, Hermes was not really what I wanted; I wanted the feelings associated with a relationship. Love, companionship, commitment, passion, safety, and adventure, all feelings one has in a relationship. If I can get attached to the feelings instead of the actual person who shows up to meet the needs, I can practice those feelings on my own.

In reality, it doesn't matter if I even have a partner, as those needs are being met, and Hermes likely wasn't the right partner anyway. They say if you want to attract a happy relationship, be happy, and the relationship will appear. So true.

I experienced significant hopelessness in life when I lost my dad, as I believed nobody could fill his shoes. That is true, nobody could. Yet this concept also created much unnecessary suffering for me, because the reality was that I was never, ever, ever going to be able to bring him back. And being attached to him in that way caused suffering for me for a very long time.

Grief is important, and key to the healing process. We must let the loss pass through us. Yet attachment is different, it is a fixation on a specific outcome, and instead of allowing myself to experience it, I ruminated on the fact that he was not here.

What I learned, with time and healing, is that I wanted father-like figures in my life to help meet my needs of love, safety, wisdom, and support from a man. So instead of wishing my father were there, I sought those people out, and found them, while also working to create those feelings in myself. The reality was, my dad didn't create those feelings, I did. His absence just inspired them.

I also learned that my focus on his absence made it harder for me to find him in my life. So instead, I focused on seeing him all around me and getting advice from him whenever I needed it. We used to always pick up pennies together, so I started associating pennies with messages from him. Was it true? It really doesn't matter. What mattered was that I got out of my feelings of sadness and into my positive feelings, where I could then be present for life.

Imagining what feelings are associated with goals really takes the concept of hope one step further. Instead of just hoping for something specific, for example straight A's, we practice and reach for feelings associated with that goal of straight A's. The feeling of accomplishment, success, growing, improving, which then opens a world of possibilities for how those desires become fulfilled.

Try that for a minute. Think of something you were recently disappointed about, something you had hoped for that you didn't attain. What was it?

Now, take a minute to think about the feeling associated with its attainment. What emotional need were you trying to fulfill? Think about that feeling. Write it down. Experience it in your body. Can you find access to it without the attainment of your goal? Is it possible? Believe it or not, you just did.

Instead of focusing on lack of it, try to think of new ways you might meet that emotional desire. Practice the experience of that emotion. I find it fascinating how often we don't even have to attain what we think we want in order to feel the way we want.

This isn't to say that attaining straight A's isn't important. Goal-setting is an important part of hope (it is the inspired actions, the second ingredient for hope), and it is important to reach for your goals. However, it is important to also understand why you are reaching for your goals and what feelings you are aiming to achieve, so that if you run into challenges or obstacles, you can use your hopeful mindset to keep moving forward.

Our program, Hopeful Minds, is a blend of the hope theories discussed along with our own interpretation and focuses on two things: how to create positive emotions and how to use inspired (and realistic) action.

We also talk about barriers to hope, or things that trip us up. We then have people create Hope Networks so they have someone positive identified to go to for support. Sometimes, though, even our Hope Networks fail us, and we have to look at awe, wonder, and faith—a connection to something bigger than ourselves.

The program itself incorporates lessons on passion and purpose, growth mindset, kindness, emotional regulation, mindfulness, gratitude, empathy, presence, intention, awe, sacredness, connection, self-efficacy, creativity, SMART goals, obstacles, change, barriers, and more.

The first thing we ask our kids is: What is hope for you? What are you hopeful about?

We have them create a personal definition, and a classroom definition, to get them working and thinking together.

I would ask the same of you. How do you define hope? What are you hopeful for? It can be one thing or many, and for various categories of your life. Are you using positive emotion and inspired action to get there? How do you want to feel when you reach your goals? Can you practice these feelings now, instead of waiting until you get there? What are you really seeking?

Consider also taking a moment to reflect on what you've hoped for recently, what goals you set. Were these 'hopes' actually attainable?

I know this is a very tough question, but are you hoping for someone deceased to return? Or are you hoping to cherish their memory, be glad you had time with them, and carry their spirit forward? I know it is easier said than done, and grief is important to healing, so it is more something to gently consider on your journey and in your time. Death has caused me so much suffering, and it has helped me to use this new perspective. Use what works for you.

Lastly, when you had a hope or a goal, were positive emotions associated with not just the destination, but the journey? Were you thinking about how you might be treating yourself, and others? Consider exploring these questions as you start to navigate your own mindset as it relates to hope.

You need only allow gentle hope to enter your heart. Exhale and allow hope and give yourself some time. This is a process of change that requires a good deal of self-compassion, which is neither stagnant nor permissive.
—Russell Brand

WHY HOPE?

To live without Hope is to Cease to live.
—Fyodor Dostoevsky

Now that we have defined hope, it is important to explore the 'why' of hope. The power of hope must not be underestimated. There is so much research around hope, and while I knew it was key to suicide prevention, I didn't realize it predicted so many other, seemingly unrelated, life outcomes.

Dr. Sanjay Gupta, in an HBO documentary *One Nation Under Stress*, looks at why life expectancy in the US is falling. As these statistics are driven primarily by an epidemic of self-inflicted deaths of despair (deaths resulting from drug overdose, chronic liver disease, and suicide), he talks about how the rise in the U.S. mortality rate can be seen as a symptom of the toxic, pervasive stress in America today.

The documentary goes on to showcase how just 4 percent of the world's population, Americans, take 80-90 percent of the world's opioids. Cyril Wecht points out that stressors like deper-sonalization, economic uncertainty, and unstable family units, coupled with self-medication or over-medication of prescription drugs, showcase the pain associated with the stress.

Is it really the stress itself, or our inability to deal with the stress effectively, that causes the deaths of despair? What is the root of it? I would argue it is our inability to create and grow hope.

Stanford neuroscientist Robert Sapolsky also featured in the documentary, studied the social behavior of baboons in the wild. He claims lack of control, lack of predictability, and lack of social support is what makes stress really corrosive. This is true for humans as well, and is exactly what we know about hopelessness and hope. And you will see all of these features—self-efficacy, navigating change, and how to create support, featured in our Hopeful Minds curriculum.

Let's look more deeply into the research on hope. We have shown, in our latest research (Kirby, 2019), that hope is in fact teachable in young children. And, in fact, as we increase hope, depression and anxiety decrease. But let's back up and look more deeply at how we got to this point.

As hope relates to mental health, one of the most encouraging studies I've found that helped reinforce the theory that hope is teachable and anxiety and depression are preventable is a study on depression, anxiety, and hope in youth (Journal of Personality, 2007). In this study, students who expressed higher hope at the beginning of the study had lower measures of depression and anxiety one and two months later. This shows that higher levels of hope can help protect one against future anxiety and depression. That is fantastic.

Even more exciting, the study revealed that the reverse **was not true**. Symptoms of anxiety and depression had no effect on future levels of hope. This indicates that if you are depressed or anxious now, it does not mean that you will be in the future.

As someone with lived experience (experience gained through direct, first-hand involvement with mental health or any particular struggles), this is exciting. It affirms that you can practice hope. You can grow these skills. Your life is not destined for anxiety and depression just because you have had it in the past.

Tell yourself, "I don't have to be a statistic. I have power over my future. It may not be easy, and it may take work, but *I have power*." This is the most exciting piece of research I have found on hope, and I have certainly found it to be true in my life.

Research also shows that hope and hopelessness are two distinct but correlated constructs. Hope can act as a resilience factor that buffers the impact of hopelessness on suicidal ideation. Inducing hope in people may be a promising avenue for suicide prevention (PLOS, 2015).

Hope also uniquely predicts objective academic achievement above intelligence, personality, and previous academic achievement (Journal of Research in Personality, 2010). Hope, but not optimism, predicts academic performance of law students beyond previous academic achievement (Journal of Research in Personality, 2011).

Hope is a strong predictor of positive emotions, and is closely related to optimism. While optimism is important to hope, it only addresses the "positive feelings" of hope, and doesn't focus on the specific "inspired actions" of hope (Journal of Positive Psychology, 2009). Hopeful people also have a greater sense that life is meaningful (International Journal of Existential Psychology & Psychotherapy, 2010).

There is also a strong business case for hope. Hopeful salespeople reach their quotas more often, hopeful mortgage brokers process and close more loans, and hopeful managing executives have a higher rate of meeting their quarterly goals (The Business Case for Hope, Forbes, 2019). Self-efficacy, optimism, resilience, and hope in the workplace are key to productivity. Hope accounts for 14 percent of productivity—*more than intelligence, optimism or self-efficacy* (Journal of Positive Psychology, 2013). Hope is a top need of employees, and effective leaders understand their followers' needs: Trust, compassion, stability, and hope. (Strengths Based Leadership, 2009)

Not convinced? To all of you sports fans out there, how about this? Hope predicts athletic outcomes. In a study of female athletes, trait hope (hope as it relates to your history with goals and success) predicted athletic outcomes; further, weekly state hope (hope in the moment) tended to predict athletic outcomes beyond dispositional hope (inherent hope), training, and self-esteem, confidence, and mood (Curry, 2007).

In a study of hope and mortality, a community sample of 1034 adults, aged 60 years and older, were evaluated, and the death data was collected within an eight-year follow-up period. In the follow-up period, the frequency of feeling hopeful, but not other individual depressive symptoms, was associated with mortality rate. The mortality rate among those who always, sometimes, and rarely felt hopeful were 21.6%, 26.4%, and 35.7%, respectively. Logistic regression also confirmed that individuals who rarely feel hopeful had higher odds of disease within the eight-year follow-up period than those who always felt hopeful, after adjusting for age and medical conditions (Zhu, 2017).

Hope is important in disease conditions and recovery as well. One study on lung cancer found that hope was inversely associated with major symptoms of cancer (Berendes, 2010). Additionally, there is evidence that individuals with greater optimism and hope seek to engage in healthier behaviors, regardless of their clinical status, and that this contributes to chronic disease treatment (Frontiers in Psychology, 2016).

This is powerful, powerful evidence for the need to focus on hope. Dr. Belfer regularly shares how his colleague, Nobel Prize winner Dr. Joseph Murray, always used a 'future orientation' with his patients. Dr. Murray did not focus on the current condition, but on what they could collectively do to create the best possible future. This is the essence of hope; inspiring positive feelings and taking inspired action.

To understand the importance of hope, we must look at the research around what it is not: Hopelessness.

This body of evidence is large, and alarming, so if you are not inspired to act on the benefits of hope, perhaps you will be motivated by the impact of not addressing hopelessness, as the costs to society are great.

Hopelessness is the leading predictor of suicide and more closely associated with suicide than depression. "Hope is the bedrock of getting out of suicidal states," says Jon G. Allen of The Menninger Clinic (APA, 2013). Hopelessness is predictive of both loneliness and suicidality, and there is no relation between loneliness and suicidality beyond hopelessness (Suicide and Life Threatening Behavior, 1996). If we want to address the global loneliness epidemic and prevent suicide, we must tackle the underlying hopelessness.

Suicide is the leading cause of death, globally, for teen girls (World Health Organization, 2008), and the second leading cause of death for all youth. Suicide rates in young girls ages 10-14 are increasing faster than boys (Jama, 2019). 1 out of 9 students are self-reporting suicide attempts before graduating high school, with 40% of them in grade school (Journal of Adolescent Health, 2011). In a recent study, 36% of adolescent girls in the US self-reported depression before graduating high school, 25% of girls in the UK before age 14, and 70% of US teens age 13-17 said that anxiety and depression are the most critical issues facing them or their peers (Pew Research Center, 2019).

This is no joke. Young kids, reportedly as young as six years old, are taking their lives. According to the CDC, a child under the age of 12 takes their life every 5 days. More than 1,300 children ages 5 to 12 have taken their own lives, and we have no idea how many have attempted. For adults, this number is estimated to be 20 times higher.

Another study points out that there are direct effects of depression and hopelessness on suicidal behaviors for males and direct effects of hopelessness and suicidal behaviors for females. This is an interesting fact as we look at gender differences between males and females, one I will explore more with the Women's Brain Project. In that same study, for both males and females, anxiety was directly linked to depression and hopelessness; drug involvement had both direct and indirect effects on suicidal behavior (Suicide and Life Threatening Behavior, 2005).

A review of hopelessness and risky behavior among adolescents living in high-poverty inner-city neighborhoods indicated the following (Journal of Adolescence, 2003):

- Adolescents react to their uncertain futures by abandoning hope, which leads them to engage in *high levels of risk behavior.*

- Of 2,468 inner-city adolescents surveyed, **nearly 50% of males and 25% of females had moderate to severe feelings of hopelessness.**

- Hopelessness predicted each of the risk behaviors considered: *Violence and aggression,* **substance use, sexual behavior, and accidental injury.**

The paper concluded that effective prevention and intervention programs aimed at inner-city adolescents should target hopelessness by promoting skills that enable them to overcome the limitations of hopelessness. Which is precisely what we are doing with Hopeful Minds.

I was about 10 when I started exhibiting addictive behavior, a time that is common for youth to start showing signs of anxiety and depression. So this was the age we initially targeted for our curriculum. My addictions began with cigarettes and alcohol, and eventually led to other substances, as a way for me to ease my discomfort with myself.

I didn't know what to do with my feelings of angst. I couldn't define my negative emotions, I just wanted to feel better. Unfortunately, our brain chemicals don't recognize the short-term difference between positive and negative experiences, so we get dopamine hits from our reward center regardless if the behavior is healthy or not. Young kids simply do not understand the difference. I sure didn't understand it, and so many adults I saw were using negative behaviors, so it seemed like a good solution.

I did what I could to feel better, with the tools I had. In turn, based on the biology of my own brain, I immediately became addicted to harmful substances. When I did something, thanks to my ADHD and focus, it was with total intensity.

What is even more concerning now is that we promote to kids a brand of 'medical marijuana.' Do you think kids know the difference between medical marijuana and street pot? Do you think they understand the impact on their developing brains? Kids across America are using pot to ease anxiety, and honestly believe it is a healthy solution. It is a real tragedy in that it creates more problems down the road.

In the mental health field, I have found that marketing and branding are often not deemed as 'respected' or 'necessary' in the research and health world, yet words matter. These kinds of decisions are critical to all kinds of outcomes, including health. I have seen the impact of negative branding on mental health. Perception is everything. It takes 50 milliseconds to make an impression, and confirmation bias (favoring information that confirms one's prior beliefs) makes changing that impression a challenge. Even something as simple as a name can have profound repercussions in society. I encourage all teams working on global mental health issues to include a branding expert who can shed light on these issues.

Smoking pot may have temporarily helped my anxiety in youth, yet it hurt my memory, motivation, and engagement in life. I can't imagine how much worse it might have been if I were seeing advertisements everywhere telling me that it was medical, legal, and healthy. Back in my day, it was illegal and frowned upon, yet I still smoked to excess to feel better.

Worse, not only did I impair my developing brain; I didn't get the therapy necessary to get to my underlying emotional issues, so I just prolonged the pain. What we avoid persists until we deal with it, especially as it relates to our emotional pain.

Though I was lucky to never have had any serious repercussions, like jail or DUIs, I am one of the few and I do not take this for granted. I had no idea I was feeling hopeless, nor did I have the tools or skills to deal with those feelings. So today, I am so committed to teaching our youth these positive skills before the age of 10, when they can more easily integrate them into their lives. The BBC documentary on Hopeful Minds shows how kids are doing this today.

Kids need to know that while substances may make them feel better in the short term, they aren't good for brain development, and don't serve them long-term. There are other, healthier options to feel better. I committed to my sobriety to teach kids it is possible to have an extraordinary life without drugs and alcohol. Identifying emotions, understanding them, and using positive coping skills are critical to eliminating hopelessness and increasing hope.

One study, in particular, showed that hopelessness is independently correlated to adolescent delinquency and violence (Maternal Child Health, 2011):

- *One in four youths (25.1%)* reported levels of hopelessness serious enough to bother them in the previous month.
- Moderate-high levels of hopelessness exhibited a statistically significant independent relationship with a range of violence-related outcomes for youth subgroups:
  - Delinquent behavior.

- *Weapon-carrying on school property.*
- All forms of self-directed violence.

This makes complete sense. If you feel hopeless, you do whatever it takes to increase dopamine and gain control and power. Unfortunately, research supports that reduced levels of dopamine lead to seeking reward in all the wrong places, including risky behavior and violence (Chester, 2016). It is hard to believe but yes, these types of thrill-seeking activities increase dopamine, the feel-good chemical of the brain.

Unfortunately, many kids may not understand that this 'feeling' is only temporary, leads to worse outcomes, and the consequences of the behaviors are negative. They don't know how harmful it is, and they are being resourceful in searching out whatever they can to feel better. Imagine how smart they would be if they were taught, young enough, the healthy ways to increase dopamine?

Senator Elizabeth Warren claims gun violence is a public health epidemic. Her website shares some pretty shocking statistics: we are now losing 100 people a day to gun violence; our firearm homicide rate in the US is 25 times higher than other comparable countries; our firearm suicide rate is nearly 10 times higher; women in the U.S. are 21 times more likely to be shot to death than women in other high-income countries, most killed by an intimate partner, and; 21 children and teenagers are shot every day.

These are terrifying and tragic statistics, and I agree we must address gun laws. In China, locking farmers' pesticides (restricting access) was an effective way to reduce suicides, as the farmers ingested pesticides lethally (means). If we look at the root cause, is gun violence really the 'health epidemic'? Or is it the feelings of extreme hopelessness that drive the behavior? I would argue that hopelessness, not gun violence, is the health epidemic and public emergency.

The statistics around hopelessness, especially in youth, are shocking. The study above shows weapon-carrying is high among hopeless youth, and 1 in 4 youth report levels of hopelessness that bother them. Think about this statistic and let it sink in—25% of youth feel hopeless on a regular basis!!

Why aren't we taking massive action to immediately increase hope and eradicate hopelessness? If hope is a better predictor of academic success than IQ, why aren't there classes on hope in school?

The percentages for lesbian, gay, or bisexual students who experienced persistent feelings of sadness or hopelessness (63.0%), and students not sure of their sexual identity with hopelessness (46.4%), as compared to the percentages of heterosexual students (27.5%) (CDC, 2018), is devastating.

How are we not making hope the norm for our youth, our workplaces, and the world? Why are we not mandating teaching this skill as part of standardized programming, when hopelessness is so often a consequence of discrimination and marginalization?

The high cost to society of not addressing hope, or addressing it much later in life, is compounding. We know hope becomes more difficult to learn the older we get, and teaching under the age of 10 is ideal, as we are finding that kids before 10 seem to integrate it into their way of being. We know that hope is a protective factor against anxiety and depression.

After 10, and when rates of depression and anxiety increase in youth, it is much harder to teach. So, another objective of our work around hope is to create a peer program developed by teens, for teens, where they teach hope to each other, informed by Hopeful Minds.

I am 100% certain I would not have listened to any of this from an adult once I got into my teen years. I knew it all, and only listened to other teens. So, my goal is to raise money to have teens create a peer-to-peer program to increase hope among themselves.

Imagine if hope was cooler than grade point average? If kids knew the importance of it, how it impacts life outcomes, and made an effort to improve it? Imagine if celebrities and leaders were creating PSAs to encourage them to do so! I imagine this every day.

The statistics around hopelessness are overwhelming. The number of things people tend to feel hopeless about only continues to grow: the environment, politics, poverty, homelessness, inequality, mental health. What is inspiring is that we can combat this sense of hopelessness by applying skills to increase our levels of hope.

Carol Dweck's work on growth mindset vs. fixed mindset has inspired my vision for Hopeful Mindsets, a way to practice the lessons of Hopeful Minds. A growth mindset is the understanding that students who believed their intelligence could be developed outperformed those who believed their intelligence was fixed. We aim to do the same with hope through Hopeful Mindsets.

We already know that hope is not a fixed trait; we have proven that it can be taught. What if we then apply it to solve global challenges, as a lot of the Hope Theory revolves around reaching goals (i.e. we might hope to end rainforest deconstruction)? This is what most excites me about the work now, because expecting to teach a child (or anyone) 16 lessons and having them automatically become hopeful is unrealistic.

However, when you start taking real-life scenarios and stories and creating a Hopeful Mindset curriculum using a blend of both, you start to see how hope applies to all aspects of life. You learn to start exercising the hope muscle, again and again and again, while learning from those who have successfully used a hopeful mindset to overcome specific challenges. This is exciting.

But back to the 'why' of hope. At this point in the book, my goal is to have convinced you that hope is key to our collective humanity. If you are not yet convinced, email me and let me know how to improve the argument or share why it isn't important. My goal is not to be right; it is to help our youth and collective humanity.

What challenges are you working on? Is hope important? How can you start incorporating the research in your work? Want to study it with us, and build on the evidence? Please do reach out.

Given the enormous role that hopelessness plays in suicide risk and in the severity of depression, teaching hope offers the vast potential to 'immunize' a whole generation of youth against suicide and depression.
—Dr. Lukoye Atwoli

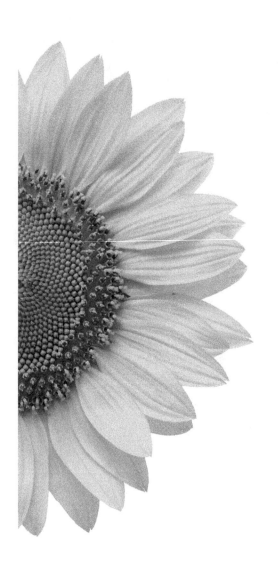

HOPE AS A FEELING

Remember, hope is a good thing, maybe the best of things, and no good thing ever dies.
—Stephen King

OUR BRAINS

You have brains in your head. You have feet in your shoes.
You can steer yourself any direction you choose.
—Dr. Seuss, *Oh, the Places You'll Go!*

In our program, we teach kids about the upstairs and downstairs brain. It is a simplistic way to look at it, but for young kids (and myself), it works.

The upstairs brain controls more complicated actions and emotions, such as decision making, self-understanding, and empathy. We use our upstairs brain to learn new things, and we enter the upstairs brain when we feel hopeful and positive emotions. It is our 'evolved' brain.

The downstairs brain controls our survival instincts. In our downstairs brain, we feel strong emotions like anger and fear—basically, our fight, flight, freeze, or fawn mode. Fight, flight, freeze, or fawn is our body's reaction to perceived danger, and the reaction of fight, flight, freeze, or fawn is our body's way to protect us from that threat. It is controlled by our downstairs brain, which can be a helpful tool when we are in trouble.

To explain this idea more thoroughly, consider a lion and a zebra. If the lion were to attack, the zebra must act quickly to either fight the lion or flee to escape the danger. The zebra could also freeze and hope the lion doesn't see it. To survive, the zebra has little time to react. It cannot stop to weigh its options.

Humans add a fourth option to the fight, flight, and freeze response: fawn. The fawn response is when you immediately try to diffuse the situation by pleasing or appeasing the other person. The fawn response is most commonly seen in people who have a history of childhood trauma.

Inside the downstairs brain, there is something called the amygdala. This almond-shaped part of the brain is powerful, as it can take control of our whole body if it senses a dangerous situation. The amygdala does this by letting the upstairs brain know that the downstairs brain suspects danger and is about to react. When the amygdala reacts, we go into fight, flight, freeze, or fawn mode.

When the amygdala and downstairs brain take over, the upstairs brain shuts down completely as our body shifts into instinct mode. Once the amygdala decides the fear or anger is over, we are often exhausted and find it hard to focus or pay attention.

As a result, if we are angry, upset, scared, or frustrated, it can be difficult to learn and retain information. It is hard to make good choices out of anger, or hopelessness, as our downstairs brain doesn't think rationally and is more violent, aggressive, combative, defensive, avoidant, or irrational. When we act while in this state, we end up creating more challenges and problems for ourselves.

While these emotions are important, they aren't effective to drive change. Think about it for a minute. When was the last time you really respected someone who was acting in moments of irrational emotions, anger, frustration, or rage? Do they motivate you? Inspire you? Is it effective?

In order to have hope, we must stay in our upstairs brain rather than letting our downstairs brain take over. There is value in 'negative' emotions, but acting from the 'positive' emotions and upstairs brain is more effective. Doing so takes practice.

Thankfully, there are tools we can use to calm our downstairs brain. These tools can help us cultivate hope inside of ourselves and be better learners, friends, family members, and successful in the future. We will be ending our lesson today by practicing one of the ways we can calm our fight, flight, freeze, or fawn response: A deep breathing exercise.

Can you remember times where you were angry, upset, or frustrated, and it seemed as if you couldn't control how you acted?

When was a time when you were able to really focus on something and remember what you learned? What did you do before that experience that may have primed your brain?

How are you feeling?

DISTRESS ASSESSMENT SCALE

Distress is any unwanted emotion, such as fear, anger, sadness, frustration, *et cetera*. Have each student rate how they are feeling on a scale of 0-10. Zero is not feeling any fear, anger, sadness, and/or frustration. Ten is feeling intense fear, anger, sadness, and/or frustration.

When our distress level reaches a 7 or higher, we may not think clearly or act in ways that are consistent with our true selves. What is your number? How are you feeling? What is your level of distress?

Students can use this tool anytime to connect with how they are feeling. When our distress reaches high numbers, self-regulation techniques may be helpful. We cover more in later exercises, but one way we can calm our mind and body is by deep breathing. (Scale provided by Dr. Elizabeth Lombardo.)

DEEP BREATHING EXERCISE

When you take a deep breath, it calms your nervous system and your downstairs brain. Any time you feel angry, overwhelmed, or stressed, taking deep breaths is important. Even if you are unable to control your reactions, you can still remember to breathe deeply. This can help you get back into your upstairs brain.

Let's practice.

1. Sit in a comfortable position with your back as flat as possible or lie on a comfortable flat surface.
2. Take a few seconds to just relax. Your neck, shoulders, arms, legs, and feet. Try a few big exhales.
3. When ready, place one hand on your chest and the other on your stomach, right below the rib cage.
4. Inhale deeply through your nose for a count of 10, if you are able, but do what is comfortable. Make sure as you breathe in, you breathe all the way to your belly. You should feel the hand on your belly rise while the hand on your chest remains still.

5. Take a moment at the count of ten, purse your lips, and slowly exhale. Feel the muscles on your stomach tighten and your hand lower.
6. Engage and notice how not just your body, but also your mind feels.

Repeat this for 5 to 10 minutes, whichever amount of time is most comfortable, and increase the amount of time spent if necessary and you are able. Practice.

What are you feeling now? Do you feel any different?

This exercise strengthens your diaphragm, and the health benefits are many. It has been shown to reduce the stress hormone cortisol in the body, lower your heart rate and blood pressure, help cope with PTSD, slow your rate of breathing, help you recover faster from exercise, and more. We encourage you to practice 2-3 times a day.

We also recommend using it when you notice your stress or anxiety levels rising. During distress, we often take shallow breaths, which puts us in fight, flight, freeze, or fawn mode and activates the downstairs brain, as it thinks there is danger. Diaphragmatic breathing helps us slow down this response to let our brains know we are okay and deactivate the stress response.

I used to be terrified of speaking. Literally, terrified. I never realized it, but I started holding my breath, and it activated this fear response. It became a vicious cycle to the point where I would have major panic attacks. However, I was able to completely shift this by using the power of deep belly breathing to assure my body everything was OK.

As such, learning the simple art of deep breathing can have a positive impact on all kinds of life experiences, not just stress. Try it before performing, presenting, speaking, singing, in the car, or any other place you might find your stress response being activated.

While those are some exercises to keep you in the upstairs brain, we also must understand the biology of our brain. Everything we do, eat, read, and 'consume' impacts how we feel. Exercise, eating the right foods, and getting out in nature, all impact our brains biology and functioning.

While we don't have 'diagnostics' yet for mental health, we are starting to make progress in understanding the 'biology' of the brain and behavior. While this book is about tools for managing states and behaviors, it by no means suggests that depression is a choice of something you can 'snap out of,' but it is something you can manage.

To illustrate this, let's look at PMS. Unfortunately, my PMS is pretty extreme, and for a few days a month, my negative filter is much stronger. I see life through a very dark filter.

This is, clearly, biology. It is likely a hormonal imbalance, and one that I wasn't even aware was an issue until I was much older. Even with Inspired Action, it is very, very difficult for me to get to positive feelings. While I can't control the feelings, I can control my awareness of what is happening, and how I act on the feelings (or don't act).

Even telling my Hope Network I am PMSing, and requesting they be extra kind, if possible, and help me reframe my thoughts, helps. I don't expect them to tolerate abuse or negative behaviors from me, yet I do appreciate compassion. So I express this, and those who love me get it.

My experience is clearly biological. There are new studies on inflammation, heart rate variability, genetics, and hormones that speak to how biology impacts our mental health. The brain is the most complex organ in the human body, and little funding has gone toward studying it, so there is still so much we don't know.

Those who debate whether it is biology or behavior miss the point; it is both. Each impacts the other, so neither needs to be 'right.' We must address both if we want to improve mental health and hope.

Medication may have saved my life, even though, at first, when I was put on it, I felt more suicidal. I knew going into it the risks of suicidal thinking, so I had my support network in place. My system eventually balanced out, and medication, coupled with intensive therapy, helped me identify and release suppressed emotions.

I'm now off all medications, and have been for five years. This has been great as well. I exercise and eat well and have cut out substances that negatively impact my biology. I make sleep a number-one priority, a key to health. If I need medication at some point, I'm not opposed to going back on it.

I'm not pro- or anti-medication, I am pro-'get informed and do what is right for you.' Just know that going on medication, without getting to the root cause of emotional imbalance, doesn't serve us. We need to do the internal work.

The impact of nutrition on the brain can't be underestimated. Have you ever noticed how different foods make you feel? We know that exercise is a powerful mood booster. What physical activities are best for your Hopeful Mindset? How do you incorporate them into your day? Try keeping a mood journal and see how your choices impact how you feel.

THE POWER OF EMOTIONS

Optimism is the faith that leads to achievement.
Nothing can be done without hope and confidence.
—Hellen Keller

I n the last lesson, we discussed emotions and acting from a hopeful place. The power of emotions and what they tell us is not to be underestimated.

For the first half of my life, I remained largely unconscious as to how I felt; I lived in survival mode and didn't know it. Sometimes I would fight and lash out, which would always make me feel worse in the end, or I would flee to escape the feelings. These reactions hurt my relationships—usually the thing I was upset about in the first place.

The reason I was so unaware of my feelings was that I was so worried all the time about how my dad felt. Was he happy? Would he be angry? What could I do to improve his mood? It didn't dawn on me that I had a right to my own feelings.

I was unaware of what was good for my brain. All I knew was that doing things that increased dopamine in my brain made me feel better. It is rewarded by both positive and negative activities.

Furthermore, my dad offered treats as a reward for things like good grades, finishing a project, or celebrating sporting events. He also did it when he messed up and felt guilty, looking to make up for his negative behaviors and moods. So, I started associating things like chocolate or ice cream with fixing emotions, based on the feeling I got from the taste and quick sugar rush, instead of talking about how or why they were there in the first place. Substances became my tool of choice to get me out of my perceived state of threat—fight, flight, freeze, or fawn—into one of serenity. Anything to increase the dopamine in my brain.

Often, when feeling a certain way, I was told I 'should not' feel that way. For example, if I did not get invited to a party, I felt sad. My parents might say, "Don't be sad, lots of other people like you." While they may mean well, it is quite normal to feel sad and left out, and okay to express it.

It became confusing to me, so I used substances to manage the confused feeling. People are meant to feel, and we all have our own experiences, and it is critical we validate the feelings of others (whether or not we agree that they should be there).

People often take others' feelings personally. As if by someone telling you how they feel when you do something, they are blaming you for it. And this may cause feelings of defensiveness in you, as you don't want to be blamed. Or you may feel that your actions have been misunderstood. However, to honor someone's feelings does not mean you have to take responsibility. But this is what often happens. And then the person gets angry that you don't see them or understand them, and the cycle continues and perhaps even escalates.

As a young and sometimes bratty teen, I would occasionally get angry at my mom for not getting me something I wanted, especially something other kids had. Was I justified for my anger or just a spoiled brat? How would you respond to me?

In my teen years, I would have argued that my anger was justified, that I was right, and that I deserved to be given what I wanted and certainly had a right to be angry.

But here is the thing, and it's where we often go wrong in relationships and feelings: Anger is a part of our human experience, and we need to recognize and honor our feelings of anger (or any other feeling) for what they tell us. Whether or not I should be angry is not the point, as our feelings and experiences of this world are valid.

If my mother reacted by shaming me or my emotions, what would that do? It would increase my anger and feelings of justification. The problem thus escalates.

I may repress the anger, hide the emotions inside me, and second-guess everything I feel because I'm told that I don't feel that way, when in reality, I do. That then eats away at my sense of self, my entire being. I question my reality.

Or I may project the anger inward, and do self-harm: develop eating disorders or cutting, anything to express or manage the pain, to the detriment of self. My anxiety and depression have always turned inward.

The end result of not learning how to effectively manage anger is that I am left with an abundance of jumbled feelings and a lack of understanding about myself. I fix the feelings with substances instead of recognizing them, listening to what they are telling me, and turning them into Inspired Action. This vicious cycle continues, ever destructive and never productive.

It is never the anger that is the issue. Rather, what we do with that anger is where we run into trouble. If I become angrier, then I'm more likely to be aggressive, abusive, unruly, disrespectful, and sure that I am right. I'm in my downstairs brain, and my mom is in hers. We have triggered each other and are escalating the issue.

The issue itself, or the goal of getting that item I want, never gets resolved. We are both acting out and harming our relationship. It is a completely unhealthy cycle that many of us regularly engage in. Worse, emotions don't go away unless we deal with them. If we repress them, they are most likely going to rear their heads again, perhaps even more loudly.

Consider an alternative reaction to the scenario. What if my mother had responded with a thought-provoking question instead of one that provoked more feelings of anger?

"I can see why you are mad that you don't get your clothes," showing understanding and presenting an opportunity to connect, so that a call to action may be heard.

"I might be angry, too," she could say, thus showcasing her empathy for me. This shows that she "sees" me.

"What do you think that anger is telling you?" This gives me an opportunity to solve my own problem while also giving me a feeling of self-efficacy. When I think about my anger, it tells me that I love that outfit, and all of the kids at school have new clothes. It tells me that I want to fit in and fear being excluded.

Anger is deeper than it looks and, in exploring this emotion, we seek out its cause. The truth of why we are angry is, in essence, a treasure map that leads to a solution. It is incredibly powerful because once we de-escalate the situation, it takes us to our upstairs brain where we can solve the problem from a positive place.

Unfortunately, I did not do this growing up. When distressed, I either lashed out or ran from the feelings, which ultimately led to chaotic relationships and a battle with addiction.

It wasn't anyone's fault. My family didn't even know I was addicted to all these substances, nor did my friends know the intensity of my pain. I was always fun; I hid it well. And as a society, we are only now just really starting to understand the power of emotions, what they can tell us, and the danger of acting from negativity.

Global research on hope supports this notion. When acting from the irrational brain space, we get unevolved actions like violence, addiction, and abuse. To change these, we must move to hope. I know my example is small and irrelevant, yet to practice emotional management is where we must start.

How can we expect kids to be hopeful if they don't understand emotions? How can we encourage kids to act from a positive place if they don't know how to get there? There is no reason to fear emotions; we must just learn how to express them.

My intense anger at the world regarding discrimination of those with mental health disabilities is massive, yet acting from this state gets me nowhere. This is true with everything. I must chunk down each and every issue, and let the anger inform me for Positive Action. I must solve what I am here to solve, little by little, using a positive framework and mindset.

Research has shown that our success at work or in life depends 80% on emotional intelligence and only 20% on intellect. While our intellect helps us to resolve problems, to make the calculations, or to process information, our emotional intelligence (EQ) allows us to be more creative and use our emotions to resolve our problems. Emotional intelligence is the ability to perceive, express, and assimilate emotion in thought through understanding the prism of emotions and adjusting our own and others' emotions (Cortrus, 2012).

I believe that learning how to act from a hopeful place is our evolution. The earth is 4.5 billion years old and humans are 200,000 years old. We are growing. If we want to live longer, we don't need higher IQs or futuristic technological advancements. To live, we need a more hopeful mindset and higher EQs.

Sadness gives us a sign that something is amiss; anger tells us people have crossed our boundaries; and happiness indicates what brings us joy. While we are only now beginning to understand them, one thing is certain: Emotions are a powerful tool.

The key is to understand the negative emotions, use them for information, and bring us to a better place for action.

What is equally powerful is when we don't just do this with ourselves, but also with others.

In the BBC documentary on Hopeful Minds in Northern Ireland, the most brilliant observation came from one of the students. He said that he noticed when his brother was upset and, instead of engaging with him at that point like he normally would (which would then result in a worse confrontation), he took a shower and went to bed. The next morning, there was normalcy and calm, a complete change in what he had experienced in the past.

He was practicing what we know as empathy. To sense and imagine the emotions of others is to practice empathy, which is a vital first step towards compassionate action, and empathy has deep roots in our evolutionary history. (Greater Good Magazine, 2020)

Cognitive and Affective empathy incites our identification and response to the emotions of people around us, be it positive feelings or those of stress, fear, or anxiety (Greater Good Magazine, 2020). Exercising empathy offers an array of benefits that may help us connect better with others. Through empathy, we may come to understand one another.

His understanding that his brother may be in the downstairs brain and being able to stay in his own upstairs brain and take a step back, led to a diffused experience and a different outcome. Empathy is important for understanding the thoughts and actions of others, as well as ourselves. This, in turn, keeps us in a place of hope.

This type of response is crucial. When other people are in their downstairs brain, they aren't acting from a rational, kind, logical place. Whenever possible, don't engage in conflict when a person is in distress. Share with them some de-escalation techniques if you think they may be open to it. Take a time-out. If you are in the middle of an argument, agree on a time to reconnect. Practice deep breathing as you engage in challenging discussions.

Some may question the simplicity of the deep breathing technique, yet its power is not to be underestimated. When you are scared, what do you do? You stop breathing. This indicates a stress response in your body. Your HRV (heart rate variability, a biological measure of stress) drops, and your body starts to panic in response to perceived threat. In this state, it is impossible to solve things rationally; you are in your downstairs brain. The breathing calms the fight, flight, freeze, or fawn response, increasing your HRV and getting you back to a better place. It is a powerful tool.

As we said at the beginning, hope is both a feeling and an action. If we want to come from a place of hope, we have to *be* in a place of hope. When angry, we take retaliatory and aggressive action when what we need is to take inspired action.

This isn't to say you should never be angry. Get angry! Feel anger. Express it in healthy ways. Find a way to release your anger, such as jogging, working out, screaming into a pillow, gardening, or even just counting to 100. Once you are back in your upstairs brain, take inspired action to respond to the situation that made you angry. If someone harms or has harmed you, seek lawful justice. If that justice is out of reach, take action to change laws standing in the way. We must cease acting from the archaic part of our brain and do the work it takes to create inspired action in order to evolve as a society.

May your choices reflect your hopes, not your fears.
—Nelson Mandela

HOPEFUL STATE PRACTICES

Where there is no hope, it is incumbent on us to invent it.
—Albert Camus

P rocessing our emotions is key to not getting them trapped in our bodies, which is where they may become future challenges. I experience PTSD (Post Traumatic Stress Disorder), not just from the death of my dad, but from early life experiences. They haunted me until I was able to remember them, process them, and release them.

Emotions can be triggered by many different things—it all depends on your past experiences and the emotions themselves, as the body and mind store these. Reaching outside of yourself can produce resources to help you navigate life's waters. You, not your emotions, are the captain.

Upon seeking aid and processing our emotions, we unlock a toolkit to help deepen our hopeful mindset. Hope is any kind of positive feeling, such as joy, abundance, clarity, creativity, pas-

61

sion, gratitude, love. These feelings allow you to create from a hopeful place.

Meditation, visualization, practicing gratitude, journaling, positive thoughts, kindness, and using creativity help us create and reinforce a hopeful state of mind. Only from stable mindsets can we move forward to our goals.

Our Hopeful State Practices rely on individual preference. Use what works for you.

The first activities are ones we can do almost anywhere and anytime. Incorporating them into our daily lives can make us more balanced and hopeful. Some of these tools may be used when your downstairs brain is knocking or has already taken over, while others can be used daily to stay hopeful over time.

DEEP BREATHING EXERCISE

For instructions on this exercise, see the Deep Breathing Exercise section of the Our Brains chapter.

This exercise is good anywhere at any time. I have used it to solve my intense fear of public speaking.

I speak regularly in front of large groups sharing very personal details of my life, and a lot of science, in front of the most brilliant scientists in the world. In the past, I would have turned red, started shaking uncontrollably, felt my throat dry up, and ultimately freeze. Thankfully, I did some work with therapists on why that happened and trained myself to anchor myself to the ground through an invisible cord summoned by deep breathing.

When public speaking in the past, my fear response would kick in from an early trauma and my breathing would automatically cease. My HRV lowered, my body went into panic. I thought

I was dying. Literally. The body does amazing things to try to save our lives.

Thankfully, deep breathing helped me tremendously to stop this cycle before it happened. To allow myself to get further and deeper into my talks, I now also think of the 'who' I am speaking for; it is never about me. It is about the millions around the world suffering, who aren't getting the support they need and deserve. I bring all of those people with me, in my mind, because I don't do it for myself—I do it for all of us. Together, still in my mind, we all breathe. It's worked miracles for me, and I hope it does for you, or someone you love who needs to share their voice and story.

But let's get back to our tools for hope. Deep breathing is one, and I cannot recommend it enough, especially with young kids (even babies). Here are a few more:

MEDITATION

As I have ADHD, I found meditation particularly challenging. Starting in a group helped, as I was too self-conscious to move around much, and the energy of the other participants calmed me.

Diving deeper into meditation, I took a class where I had to meditate two hours a day. This was where I figured out how to get my mind to quiet. I practiced this for four months and, initially, it took me roughly 45 minutes to reach that place of silence. Today, I can get there right away.

Meditation has been found to enhance memory, improve creativity, reduce anxiety, increase relaxation, promote better sleep, lower blood pressure, and aid emotional well-being. There are many great apps and online sources for meditation. Insight Timer is a free app where you can set the amount of time to meditate and use guided meditations. YouTube has tons of free videos. Feel free to explore.

Personally, my biggest benefit from meditation has been to quiet the mind so that I am not micromanaging everything in my world. My mind responds to situations with fearful action, the downstairs brain, in situations where allowing things to happen organically would result in my decisions stemming from inspired action.

Meditation enables the mind to slow negative emotions like fear and promotes a peaceful mindset. It helps train us to be able to do that in real life. If we are in a stressful situation, it becomes easier to let the thoughts float by without triggering the downstairs brain. It is an incredible tool, and I hope you find a method that works for you.

This is what we encourage teachers to do with students: Have students get as comfortable as possible. It is okay if students remain in their seats/desks for this activity, but the classroom needs to be as quiet as possible. This activity takes five minutes.

- Have students close their eyes, keep their bodies still, and focus only on breathing. As you breathe in and out, through your nose when possible, focus on the sensation of air right between your lips and nose.
- When your mind wanders, focus on the breath and the sensation right below the nose.
- If it is helpful when they are beginning, students may count to five in their head as they inhale and count to five again as they exhale. The goal is to quiet their mind/thoughts, be still, and focus only on each breath.

VISUALIZATION

We often create without intention and then wonder why our lives are a mess. Creating for the sake of creating, without understanding what we really want or what it may produce, is to act without drive. As if on autopilot, we make new products for the sake of new products and enter meetings simply because they are scheduled. Rarely do we consider why we do these things. What outcome are we seeking?

Visualization, forming mental images of the future you want, helps you connect to your intentions. It allows you to recognize your wants and enables you to take those feelings into your body, so that you may better understand your goal. Visualization can be a useful tool to use before a date, meeting, vacation, or family event. Taking time to visualize yourself acing a test or playing a perfect game the night before can actually increase your success.

Want to practice visualizing a positive outcome for something in your life? Take a second to get settled. Close your eyes and focus on something coming up that you want to turn out well. Think about its perfect scenario. Continue to focus on this positive image for 30 seconds (or as long as possible) and notice the sensations you feel in your body. Breathe deeply and consider how the outcome is created. Then, take a few minutes to appreciate the time taken to visualize a positive outcome. Let this positivity impact your world.

PRACTICING GRATITUDE

Happiness is not having what you want,
it is wanting what you have
—Sheryl Crow

For long-term distress, consider the gratitude technique. Even on the worst of days, the days where you feel there is nothing good left, try to find something to be grateful for, anything.

Make gratitude a daily practice. Keep in mind three things every day for which you are grateful, so that you can start shifting your focus to what is good in life. This gratitude helps you stay hopeful even if there are events out of your control that challenge your hope.

- Make a mental list of things you appreciate.
- Select a time to declare three things you are grateful for every day.

To have productive and healthy relationships, we need to say five positive things for every negative thing. If you are having trouble with a coworker or friend, look at how many criticisms you are making compared to appreciations. It needs to be a 5:1 positive to negative ratio. The results may surprise you.

JOURNALING

Express emotions by getting them out of you and onto paper. Journaling helps empty the mind, which is ideal during stressful times. If you are overwhelmed with tasks, even writing them down on paper may help ease worry. Or writing about what the emotions would say to you if they had a voice.

This is especially helpful at night if you are lying awake worrying. If you find yourself in your head, lying in bed unable to shut off your mind, take a few minutes to write down what you are thinking about. That act can help put your mind to rest so you can get a great sleep.

There are many forms of journaling, but a very simple one is simply writing down positive things that happened throughout your day. No matter how big or small, find something that makes you smile. If you can't think of anything, try to remember the last time you felt joy. Write about that joy.

While it is often cathartic to write about the negative feelings, remember to let them inform you. What are they telling you? Are there any positive actions you can take? Do what you can to end on a good note.

CREATIVE ACTIVITY

Relax your emotions and prepare your brain for hope by doing activities that are creative. Playing music, using your imagination to make up skits or stories, coloring, drawing, photography, designing other art projects, or any other activity where you use your creativity, can help you release tension, anger, stress, and frustration in order to prepare you for a mindset for hope.

FORGIVENESS

We cannot be hopeful with anger in our hearts. And lack of forgiveness has been shown to have negative health effects. Everett Worthington, Jr. has studied the Science of Forgiveness, and has published many papers on the impact of unforgiveness on the immune system and overall health. Ruminating about something others have done is harmful, and we feel a lack of control or self-efficacy.

Forgiving, on the other hand, has been shown to have a number of positive health benefits. The what and how of forgiveness is a much longer book, yet I thought it important enough to bring up here as it is a critical skill for hope. We explore this further in our curriculum, and with our kids.

In the meantime, you may want to consider if there are people in your life you haven't forgiven. And start learning from places like Psychology Today, or The Greater Good Science Center, on ways you might go about thinking of forgiveness in your life.

KINDNESS

November 13th is World Kindness Day, yet we suggest you practice kindness every day. Kindness can be in a simple gesture or giant act. Big or small, each act of kindness helps make the world a better place. Here are some suggestions for kindness:

- Smile at a stranger. Smiling releases endorphins, the feel-good chemical in the brain. See if you can inspire a smile from them.
- Compliment someone. Be specific.
- Plant a tree or sunflower.
- Host a fundraiser for someone in need.
- Visit a retirement center.
- Volunteer at a soup kitchen.
- Mentor a student.
- Volunteer for a hotline.

Opportunities are limited only by your imagination. The sky's the limit. As you are kind to others, notice not just how it makes them feel, notice how it makes you feel.

Kindness is not an afterthought... It is the driving power for everything... To me, almost every problem you can think of can be solved with kindness. At least it could be made better.

—Lady Gaga

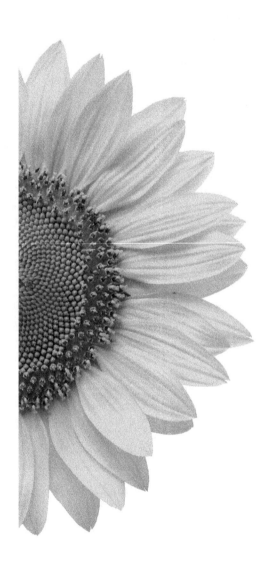

HOPE AS AN INSPIRED ACTION

The best way to not feel hopeless is to get up and do something. Don't wait for good things to happen to you. If you go out and make some good things happen, you will fill the world with hope, you will fill yourself with hope.
—Barack Obama

SMART GOALS

To be without hope is like being without goals,
what are you working towards?
—Catherine Pulsifer

The Biggest Little Book About Hope has, so far, addressed the "feeling" part of hope. Now, we are going to focus more on "action" by looking at goals, agency, and pathways. Here are some key guidelines for goals:

- Identify realistic goals
- Set stretch goals for your long-term purpose, and then chunk it down into smaller, more manageable goals
- Be able to define S.M.A.R.T. Goals:
  - Specific
  - Measurable
  - Achievable
  - Relevant

- ▪ Time-Bound
- Set small goals / micro-goals to make progress
- Ensure that your goals are achievement goals, not avoidance goals
- Celebrate each step achieved along the way
- Enjoy the journey

Goals are such an important part of hope, yet who teaches us how to set smart goals as kids? Do we ever set realistic goals? This is so key to hope.

Achievable goals are the first step to self-improvement.
– J.K. Rowling

We often ask kids at this stage what success is to them. They come up with being a doctor, lawyer, musician, and so on. While these are great ambitions, is this really the purpose of life? Most doctors, lawyers, and musicians would say no.

We place so much emphasis on the attainment of goals, the success phase, that we don't enjoy the journey it takes to reach that destination. Oftentimes, we may treat others poorly in order to reach that "success" faster, only to finally arrive and find it unfulfilling, if not empty.

Goals are tools for having hope because they give us something to look forward to and encourage us to work toward our future. We can enjoy the steps we take to get there and feel a sense of accomplishment along the way. Success is enjoying the journey and treating yourself and others in a way that makes you proud regardless of whether you reach the destination.

Our goals may change over time, or we may fail in achieving them. Our ability to navigate this change determines how hopeful we remain. Thankfully, we can always set new goals.

In order to use goals as hope tools, we must set realistic goals. By outlining all the specific action steps we need to take in order to help ourselves move forward, our goals remain realistic.

Action steps are pathways that help take us to our goal. With each step, we can feel a sense of fulfillment and enjoy each success along the way.

Think of winning the lottery. Many people say they "hope" to win the lottery, but is this an effective way to use hope? What specific steps would you have to take and what is the likelihood you would actually win?

If you spend all of your savings on the lottery or some other game of chance to the point that you can't pay your bills and lose your home, how hopeful are you going to be? That is how a false hope can pave the road to destruction and lead you down a trail of hopelessness. The importance of realistic goals cannot be stressed enough; it is why we need a rebranding of hope, as it is often misused in everyday life.

One way we can achieve realistic goal-setting is by creating a S.M.A.R.T. goal. This tool can help create a plan to improve our chances of reaching goals and acquiring a sense of accomplishment.

THE MEANING OF S.M.A.R.T.

Specific: Who needs to be involved? What are you trying to accomplish? What is your timeframe? Where is the location? Which requirements may be involved? Why do you want this goal? How much will it cost? Can you afford it?

Measurable: Do you have a way to measure your progress? Consider setting milestones if it is a goal that may take time to reach.

Achievable: Does your goal inspire motivation within you? Do you have the tools or skills you need? Do you have the money and resources? Do you have people who can help? If not, do you know how to obtain them?

Relevant: Does your goal make sense with what you are trying to achieve? Does it fit with your passion and purpose?

Time-Bound: Is your timing realistic? Can you achieve your goal in the time period you've set? Think about what you may want to achieve at the halfway point. If possible, set micro-goals along the way and celebrate your progress.

Think of a goal you have been wanting to achieve. Are you achieving it? How can you use this framework to support you in the process?

It does not matter how slowly you go
as long as you do not stop.
—Confucius

In order to use your goals as hope tools, it is okay to set small goals and work toward them slowly. Every goal you achieve helps you stay hopeful. Setting big goals is exciting but accomplishing the steps along the way is just as important. Celebrate each success.

This is one of my hardest challenges in life. My ADHD was not diagnosed until I was in my late 30's. One of the beautiful things about ADHD is the ability to hyper-focus, which allows me to see a goal and go after it. It is amazing!

On the downside, my brain doesn't care as much about enjoying the journey. It sees the end goal and wants it done. I'll sit down for 10 hours, so completely absorbed in my task that I don't get up to get exercise, eat nutritious foods, or call my friends to say hello. My brain sees these activities as wasteful and inefficient because I am trying to get something done.

The problem is that that way of operating is devastating to my mental health. The isolation from people kills me; the lack of exercise lowers my endorphin levels; the lack of nutrient-rich food depletes my brain and body. How is this creating a hopeful mindset? It isn't.

Yet my brain works most efficiently this way. It sits down and gets going and can't be interrupted. I can't tell you how many flights I've missed because I have gotten there too early and then become absorbed in a task. It happened last week.

I've had to learn how too much absorption in a task negatively impacts my projects and relationships, ruins the fun of the journey, and has a negative impact on my mental health. I've had to realize that my work won't get done in my timing and that, instead, it will get done in the universe's timing.

I must savor the nutrition I put in my body for what it does to my brain and make exercise my number one priority. My mental health suffers greatly if I don't. I also make sure to work in no more than 3-hour chunks, then do something else for at least 30 minutes, when possible. I take extended time off when I need it. And I try, at minimum, to get up every hour and stretch when I am at my computer. I've still got to figure out the airport thing.

By setting small goals along the way, taking small breaks, and making sure exercise and nutrition are my number one priority, I can reach my goals and enjoy the process every step of the way.

What goals do you have? Are your goals SMART? Are there goals you are putting off? What micro-goals can you set to start achieving them?

Are you pairing positive emotions with the goals? Celebrating small successes? Taking care of your emotional and brain health along the way?

PASSION AND PURPOSE

> *We dream to give ourselves hope. To stop dreaming, well,*
> *that's like saying you can never change your fate.*
> —Amy Tan, *The Hundred Secret Senses*

A vital component of a strong hope foundation is knowing that you have meaning and value. We all are important and add great value to the world. Not one of us on this planet is without a purpose, if only every child and adult realized it.

People who uncover their passions and purpose are often happy and fulfilled. Pursuing your purpose makes you more hopeful, even though you may deal with challenges along the way. You can begin to uncover your purpose by recognizing what you enjoy.

Our purpose is often something we are passionate about (something you love or find meaning in doing) that intersects with what you are good at doing.

Ask yourself these questions:

- What is one thing that you know you enjoy doing?
- What do you love to do?
- What activities excite you?

We teach kids that art, friendship, taking care of animals, writing stories, running a business, or building things might be their purpose, and that there is no purpose better than another. What is important is that they think about what they are good at and what they enjoy. We want them to pursue these things.

Ambitious from a young age, my first lemonade stand sold toys, candy, and things I found people might want to impulse-purchase. I bought them at the local candy store and resold them at 3x the cost. Who could resist a young child? I worked not because I needed the money, but because I was fascinated by commerce and I loved the art of business.

I went on to run canteens, wash dishes, and work at a record store, always making sure that I had a job or two. I wanted to be a waitress when I grew up, yet it wasn't my strong suit—I couldn't remember anything—so I stuck to retail. Anytime I did research, created processes or efficiencies, or implemented strategies, I thrived.

My dad was a retail banker and brought my brother and me to work on Saturdays and Sundays. Awed by the tall steel curved tower, I remembered the sounds of the "L" train clanking as we headed down to his bank in Chicago. Dad told us endless stories about how Sam Walton was going to change the world with retail.

When my dad and I traveled (as we often did to our farm in Wisconsin), he would take me into stores looking for empty shelves while talking about how Sam's revolution of "Just in Time" inventory was going to change the face of retail. According to him, there wouldn't be wasted costs in the back-storage areas, it would save money for all, and people would get products sooner.

He told me about the sure success Walmart would have, and he celebrated that success every day. My brothers and I pitched

Walmart to each of our investment classes in high school, and my brothers and I all won.

Equal to my love for retail was my love for humanity. I'd volunteer at soup kitchens, mentor kids in math, and save animals that needed homes. When my parents argued, I could not sit still and let them be, I would jump into the middle of the argument and try to resolve it. When anyone picked on my brothers, I would jump right in (much to my brothers' dismay). I had to step in. This empathy for others ran so deep that I considered it both a blessing and a curse.

So, growing up with this retail background, and having a compassionate heart, I started deeply wondering why so many consumer products companies simply launched new flavors, sizes, or styles. There never seemed to be a purpose other than profit behind new products, and this really perplexed me. I wanted both products and purpose.

This started to get addressed through 'Cause Marketing', i.e.: companies launching products while raising money for a cause. They were at least doing good with their new laundry detergent. Their Inspired Action made me happy.

Yet I felt there was still something missing. These products still seemed to be launched just to get something new to the market and weren't driven by a greater need to do good. I believe this frustration was the beginning of my seeds for The Mood Factory and iFred, yet I still didn't really know it.

These were all rather fleeting thoughts, however. As I spent the first 30 years of my life focusing on being 'liked', with the primary purpose of work to be productive and useful to others while using substances to distract me from myself. There would be moments of sobriety and clarity, yet they didn't last long. Those years in addiction kept me apart from my true purpose. Thankfully, I continued to build skills that later served my purpose, so it wasn't a total waste.

At a time when I was clear-headed, I wrote a paper for my MBA class with a mission statement that said I was here to create a social impact company and a nonprofit. I had no recollection of this. So, when cleaning out my old files, and finding the paper 15 years later, you can imagine my surprise. I believe we all know our purpose deep within, we just have to sit still long enough to discover it.

Nothing is more frustrating than not being able to pursue your purpose, especially once it has been found. I've almost destroyed my company a few times due to unhealed issues and my desire to help others before helping myself, a pattern I carry over from childhood. I've gone against my instincts, not listened to my inner voice, and put others' projects before mine because of limiting beliefs about my own value. I've worked to release these, as the truth is, we each have our own purpose. While we can support others, it is important to believe in and focus on our own stories.

A purpose doesn't have to be some massive passion project. As a society, we so often forget what makes us all tick. What allows things to run smoothly is each other. The cleaners, the electricians, the teachers, the businesspeople, the politicians, the moms, the grandfathers, the crossing guards—every person has a role in making our community work.

Everyone needs to feel their meaning and purpose; it is a key ingredient of hope.

There are many books on finding your purpose, yet I learned one simple exercise that helped me solidify it. It meant looking at my deepest pain, the thing that hurts me more than anything in the world. What did that pain tell me? From pain, comes passion, which can be channeled to purpose.

Before charging ahead, it is important to do the healing work around it. You can be certain, when I was furious about my father's death, I was not a shining star for hope or happiness. It is really only through 15 years of deep work in sobriety, intensive therapy, and taking care of myself first and foremost that I am in alignment. As we have stated, we aren't effective at working from negative emotions. Yet this pain can serve as fuel for action.

What is your greatest pain? How might you use it to serve humanity? Have you found your purpose? Do you feel you are living your life's mission?

If you find yourself stuck, consider making a list of things you are passionate about. Journal about different paths you could take in your life based on what you love. Dream about how it might be to pursue these passions.

You can also consider examining your strengths, and how they may help you to find your purpose. You can learn more about your strengths by taking the VIA Character Strengths Survey at https://www.viacharacter.org/survey/account/register.

Think about how it would feel, where you would live, and the people who would be with you. An abundance of resources are available, be they in person or online. All you have to do is begin looking, and you are well on your way to hope.

One of the most painful experiences in my life was when my dad died. However, this is also the experience that led me down my current life journey. I realized that I didn't want anyone else to die by suicide, and I made it my mission to understand why suicide occurred and how it could be prevented. This became my purpose, and led to iFred, Hopeful Minds, and my research on hope and hopelessness.

SURRENDER

> *Sometimes, you have to stop trying to force it;*
> *walk away and let your subconscious show you the way.*
> *Fill up on life for a while.*
> —J.K. Rowling

My favorite book in the world is *The Surrender Experiment* by Michael Singer. It changed my life. I always thought 'meditation-type people' were not of the business world, and that you could not accomplish great things through surrender. Michael Singer is living proof this is not the case.

Self-tasked with fixing everyone else while unable to practice any form of surrender led to a lot of my mental health challenges earlier in life. Growing up, I could not sit in negative feelings, and those led to impulsive actions (as opposed to Inspired Actions). So I often did way, way, way more work than required, simply because I wasn't acting from a positive place.

What I didn't know was that surrender is not a lack of action. Rather, it is *inspired action*. To surrender is to take in all the information with grace and ease, and act with purpose from a relaxed positive mindset. A kind of knowing. I was a doer, but I was anxious and depressed and addicted and exhausted by my doing, as it was often driven by fear rather than inspiration.

Once I sobered up and reconnected with my initial purpose (happiness) as an adult, and practiced that feeling again and again,

I launched Mood-lites with a Cause Marketing component. I cared less about my destination and more about my journey. I got serious about my recovery, got in therapy and on medication, did deep healing work, and surrendered to my journey, accepting that I am who I am. I didn't need to be anyone or anything else.

A few years into my company and nonprofit, I made the difficult decision to leave my marriage. Burdened with significant debt, I decided that instead of engaging in a battle, I would release my ego and focus 100% on getting my mental health in order. I would surrender.

This was one of the most significant lessons of my life, as I had to completely release my need to be 'right' and practice extreme self-care. The ego has a strong need to be 'right.' It used to think that if I didn't engage and didn't prove my point, it meant I was weak. I now know the opposite.

Divorce is incredibly painful, no matter what the situation. I wanted to stay married, yet I found that as I got sober, I became more sensitive to the energy around me. And I took care of others, often at the expense of myself. I really needed to learn how to hear my own needs, and how to take care of myself.

So, I sat with profound sadness, as I had run my company and nonprofit into the ground. I viewed it as my purpose, and saw no way out. My hopelessness was high. I tried in vain to take back control and save both, yet I was in over my head and had no more options. I knew the only truly important thing in life was to get my mental health back on track, not to care so much about the 'external factors'. I needed to stop running and learn to just be.

So, I surrendered and relinquished all control, focusing only on my mental health, ignoring my business and nonprofit. I literally gave up on it, got to therapy three times per week, got on the right medication, surrounded myself with family, worked out every day (even if it was just slow walking), meditated, wrote, spent time in nature, fostered animals, sang in a choir, and surrendered to any attachment of success with my company and nonprofit. I did only what brought me joy and released my pain.

I put my positive mindset and emotional state first. I practiced complete and total surrender. It was only then that things turned around.

Led by the universe and my own inner voice, which I was finally starting to hear, my company and nonprofit took off. I got an appointment to talk to a buyer at Lowe's and shared with them a vision of a lighting set that had a Cause Marketing campaign strategy. The buyer introduced me to the Public Relations (PR) team, and I shared with them the celebrities who were engaged, and the extensive press coverage on my work to date, and my vision for nonprofit activation.

We sold 9 million Mood-lites, doubled their SKU x SKU sales, and grew the colored lighting category significantly. I paid off my debt, did the first nationwide Cause Marketing campaign for hope (also raising money for breast cancer, autism, and heart disease), and got my life back on track. I stopped depending on others for my happiness and started creating my own.

The Surrender Experiment, followed by a reflection on my own life, provided living proof that making decisions from a place of calm, ease, and hope, as opposed to anger, fear, and ego, led to great success. I was that living proof.

I truly had to let go of control, of any attachment to outcome, make my mental health and emotional state a number one priority, and allow myself to be guided for everything to change for the better. Clearly, I am not perfect in this, as I have had slips. Yet, as with everything, I seek progress, not perfection.

I want you to think about that for just a minute, as it truly goes against everything we have ever learned about success. I was taught to go after it aggressively. Yet it is only when I stopped doing this that it came easily. This astounded me.

So why is surrender vital to hope? Surrender gives us the time and space necessary for hope to grow.

How might you apply surrender to your own life? Are there places where you are 'pushing too hard'? Are there ways you might step back and let things unfold? Try even a small step in that direction to test the theory and see what happens.

OBSTACLES TO HOPE

Hope is a beautiful thing. It gives us peace and strength and keeps us going when all seems lost. Accepting what you cannot change doesn't mean you have given up hope. It just means you have to focus your hope on more humanly tangible and attainable goals.
—Julie Donner Andersen,
What My Widowed Husband Has Taught Me

CHANGE AND THE PIVOT

Hope is like a road in the country; there was never a road,
but when many people walk on it, the road comes into existence.
—Lin Yutang

In order to keep ourselves hopeful, we must learn how to deal with change. Obstacles to our goals arise and, sometimes, goals have to change. Our ability to be flexible in this enables us to enjoy our journey and remain in a hopeful place.

I would not have chosen this path to hope if I weren't divinely inspired. This divine inspiration is something deep within me that, when I am really silent, tells me that this challenging yet rewarding path is my journey.

I am also certain I would not have chosen to run my company, The Mood Factory, and nonprofit, iFred, at the same time. One is hard enough. Yet when I tried to convince other nonprofits to change their branding for mental health, they didn't agree. And when I see a problem that needs fixing, I am not one to sit idle.

It is also difficult to keep the memory of how I lost my dad alive through my advocacy work. Many days, I would prefer to forget the whole thing. Yet I am certain he would have wanted me to share this knowledge with others. And I believe when all is said and done, he will not be remembered for how he died, but for his eternal quest for happiness and hope and wish for others to have it.

So, when I cry in frustration at the world's inability to understand me and the overwhelmingness of all the challenges, the deep knowledge within me lifts me up. When I feel I have no more solutions for how to manage and grow both my company and nonprofit without destroying myself, solutions appear. This divine inspiration, or purpose, is my driving force.

Entrepreneurs have a high rate of depression. Take into consideration the obstacles that must be overcome in order to reach a destination, the number of 'no's' we hear, the number of failures. The unforeseen circumstances attempting to affect progress are an ongoing avalanche of pivots, solutions, modifications, and barriers.

These obstacles, however, are challenges that we can navigate. It is our ability to overcome challenges, or what Snyder and Hope Theory refers to as Create Pathways, which allows us to remain hopeful. We must have the flexibility necessary to adapt.

When we set our goals or consider our passion and purpose, it is helpful to envision what might get in the way. Imagine the many circumstances that may prevent you from achieving your objective, but don't let them deter you. Know thy enemy and be educated, so that you can adapt.

For instance, your child wants to go to college. What obstacles might they face? Grades, money, distance, homesickness, *et cetera*. Ruminating on the problems ahead of time can help you develop solutions for potential challenges (saving, studying more, therapy, friends).

What goals are you currently setting for yourself? Have you thought about the challenges you might face along the way? Are you prepared for them?

I think one of the hardest things about goals is knowing when to let them go. Running a company and a nonprofit at the same time, totally bootstrapped, puts me under incredible pressure. I don't currently have the big budget, infrastructure, or support staff I had at a place like American Express, so I must be flexible and adaptable. I often ask myself, is this it? Is it time to walk away, close up shop, and call it a day?

And I ask for divine guidance. I go outside for a hike, meditate, and do the next inspired thing. I don't ask for answers now, I just make the next best decision that is in front of me. I become present and know that all will be revealed.

I don't have the resources to rewrite the curriculum, and I'm frustrated by it, so I get my frustration out with exercise and form the idea to write the book, to share what I know about it, and surrender to the situation.

Will writing this book really matter? Who knows? It doesn't really matter (nonattachment to outcome, and surrender). What is important to me is that I feel good doing it, it allows me to clarify my vision, and it comes from divine inspiration. It meets my need for hope through feeling positive and acting from an inspired place. And it allows me to share with others in a practical way what I know, which is why I do this work.

So every day, I use this mindset with this work. If I need to pivot, I know it will not destroy me. Many people change their goals due to unforeseen circumstances, and it is their ability to do so that predicts their capacity for hope. I will let that same grace take me on the hope-and-mood journey, or a new journey, whatever it may be. I don't have to know now if I need to let it go, I just need to take the next step.

Many people, upon retirement, experience depression because they find that they have lost their purpose. The reality is our purpose in life may change. Our purpose may become being a friend, or grandmother, or just to make someone smile. It is our ability to navigate these changes, and remain in a positive state, that ensures our ability to remain hopeful.

If you are wondering whether to give up and walk away on a specific project or vision, I implore you to look at your own mental health and the health of those around you. Are you taking care of yourself? Are you feeling your best?

Are you bringing out the best in others? Is your daily inner experience reflected in your work? If you give it all up and walk away, what happens? How do you feel? Does it follow you?

That's where you will find your answer.

However bad life may seem, there is always something you can do and succeed at. Where there's life, there's hope.
—Stephen Hawking

WORRY AND ANXIETY

*Hold your head high, stick your chest out. You can make it. It
gets dark sometimes, but morning comes. Keep hope alive.*

—Jesse Jackson

Unmanaged worry leads to anxiety, which then leads to a state
of panic. Worry is in the mind, which is usually preoccupied
with a future event that may or may not come to be. This
emotion is often incredibly unhelpful, as it keeps us out of the
present moment.

My panic attacks from speaking came from worry. A thought
would come to my mind and I'd worry over tiny details, which
led to the emotion escalating. My breaths arrived in short bursts
before stopping entirely, alerting my autonomic nervous system. In
a panic, I'd sit frozen throughout a meeting, all from worry.

Worries keep us up at night, keep our system in a state of high
alert, and are wasted energy since they aren't in our control. Letting
worry take you into a state of stress and anxiety is an ineffective use

of the emotion. An effective use of worry is to attach it to a smart goal and find a solution.

My public speaking anxieties escalated to worrying constantly about speaking, presentations, and conversations. Stressing for days, I'd escape through my addictions and do everything possible to avoid situations where I would have to speak.

Everything changed when I learned how to start breathing and become present.

One of our biggest challenges in life is maintaining a state of presence. Practices like meditation and mindfulness help us calm our minds, but how do we really engage in life? How can we not just be in our bodies, but become more active participants? How could I take what I learned in meditation and apply it to life?

One of the easiest ways to become present is to engage the senses (Stern, 2004).

If I am speaking about an emotional subject and feel myself welling up with tears, I breathe through and give myself a moment. It has been 30 years, and I still cry about my dad when I talk. I miss him so much. I want him here, helping me with my business. I need his financial expertise, as that was his brilliance.

However, when I feel my mind taking over, again leaving the present and letting my thoughts run wild, I anchor back down into the present. I use my breath and the senses of smell, touch, sight, sound, or taste to anchor myself. I hold onto the podium. I feel my feet on the floor. I anchor myself in the present.

Recall something you're worried about: bills, health, relationship issues, or something else. Upon thinking of that worry, how does your heart react? How does your body feel? Where do you feel it?

If you find yourself getting upset at the thought, touch something, right now. Feel it and explore the sensations. Focus on that feeling. You can also try it with scent, sound, taste, or sight. Do what feels best.

Doing that small exercise may bring you to a place where you are not thinking about the past or the future—you are in The Now. Intercept the trigger before it happens. Kill the worry with your senses.

According to Jon Kabat-Zinn, creator of the *Stress Reduction Clinic and Center for Mindfulness in Medicine, Health Care, and Society* at the University of Massachusetts Medical School, mindfulness means paying attention to the present moment, on purpose and without judgment. It takes work to get into the present. While meditation helps us achieve calming the mind and easing worry, how can we also truly engage in The Now?

A famous Harvard study showcased that we are out of the present moment almost 50% of the time with our wandering minds. The study further showed that we always feel worse, no matter what we are thinking about, when our mind is wandering. We are happiest and most engaged when in the present moment (Science, 2010).

When we are happy and engaged, our dopamine levels rise and our minds work better. With our brains engaged, we are more likely to collaborate, produce, create, solve problems, help others, and participate in physical activities (Diamond, 2009). When we get pleasure and satisfaction from activities that generate positive feelings, we are less likely to seek pleasure from high-risk, detrimental activities (Galván A et al, 2006).

Research suggests, instead, that being present and in a state of flow is when people are at their happiest (Chentmihalyi, 1997).

Flow is a state of mind where a person gives his or her undivided attention to the task at hand, senses fully immersed for intrinsic reasons. We believe that, when all of us start living in the here and now, we will all be much happier, healthier, more productive, and better contributors to society.

One of the easiest ways to engage in The Now is through sensory engagement. Research also suggests that the more senses you engage in the right way, the more intense your experience (Gottfried and Dolan, 2003).

Consider sleeping, for example. You can lie on a bed and sleep. Yet if you really want to create an incredible experience of sleep, you need the sounds, scents, touch, taste, and sights (or lack thereof) to be in alignment for sleep. If you have trouble sleeping, try looking at each of these areas and seeing where you can modify them to create the perfect sleep.

When enjoying a delicious cup of tea, how can you savor the experience? The answer with tea is easy: Drink slower, inhale the fragrance, notice the flavor, i.e.: take more meaningful sips. And what of the world around us? How can you savor your day-to-day experience as much as possible?

What about meditation? Deep breathing? Do we really have more problems, or are we just being lazy about our moods and how we experience life?

Do we focus on what we love, or what we hate? I always hated the glass-half-empty analogy, yet it is true that if we look at the half glass empty, that is what we see in life. And if we look at the half glass full, that is what we see as well. Many new analogies have come up as well, so we have to be aware of our perception, and make sure it is positive.

A positive outlook takes diligence, work, and practice to focus on what we love. Happiness and hope are both skills. So is stress. We have trained ourselves to be stressed. We can manage it just fine if we want to, yet again and again we choose the easy way out—smoking, drinking to excess, overeating, gambling, crime, shopping, and other unhealthy activities and quick fixes.

What do we teach our kids to focus on, to savor? Their worries and fears, or what they enjoy and delight in? Research is showing us our kids are more stressed than we are, but who is it they are emulating? It is time for us all to relearn the joy of presence.

How does presence relate to hope? We can't maintain a sense of hope if we aren't experiencing the moment and are instead living in a state of stress and anxiety. By using presence techniques when we find our minds wandering, we are brought back to the here and now. We can't get to a place of hope if we come from a place of worry. Presence keeps us grounded and happy.

It works brilliantly with kids in class. During one of my hope talks last year, the kids were all over the place. Fidgeting, restless, looking around. I could tell their minds were miles away, so I asked them what they smelled.

The simple act of smelling and breathing deeply through the nose brought them back to the present moment. It allowed me to then guide them into the actual lesson I was trying to teach, as they were engaged, participating, and listening. You can do this exercise with any of the senses.

Think about it. Which of your sensory experiences do you most enjoy? Are you a fan of sight, sound, taste, touch, or smell? Think about how different sensory experiences make you feel.

Now think of an event that stressed you out. What can you control in this environment? What can you influence to bring more joy to the experience?

What are you teaching your kids? How can you inspire them to be more in the moment?

FAILURE

When the world says, 'Give up,'
Hope whispers, 'Try one more time.'
—Vikrmn

A t a young age, for whatever reason, I thought I was my dad's therapist. His mental health was untreated. If he felt angry, I tried to fix it. If he felt sad, I did everything I could to make him happy. I walked on eggshells a lot of the time.

When I lost my dad in college, I was devastated. For every negative quality about him, there was an equally amazing positive. He was fun, gregarious, loving, generous, smart, successful, yet burdened with years of untreated pain that he projected outward.

In seconds, after years of me trying to save his life, he was gone. His life was over. He chose the final escape. He completely gave up hope that he could ever be happy.

One of the hardest lessons I learned was that I could not make my dad hopeful or happy. I could not save him. I could not convince him I was worth sticking around for. And believe me, I tried.

When my dad died, not only did I lose one of the most important people in my life, but I also considered myself a failure. Rationally, I knew it wasn't my fault, but I internalized the loss more than those around me. I was coming home that weekend from Iowa to spend the weekend with my dad. He was let out of the hospital early and was alone in a large house. If only I had been there…

This is what happens in the minds of many who have lost a loved one to suicide. I've talked to so many. The 'if only' scenarios we play over, and over in our minds. Yet I also know, unequivocally, we are not to blame.

I know, because if I had died by suicide, it would have been my fault, and my fault only. I'd gotten myself to that state. I was the one who had made the choices leading up to it.

I knew of resources, yet chose not to use them. 'I got this.' I prioritized pleasure over pain. I never thought it would go there. While someone may be able to fix my temporary problem, if I haven't fixed the root cause, the problem will come back in another way. Trust me.

And even today, my decisions are my own. Even knowing everything I know, there is still a chance I might die by suicide. There is nothing anyone can do to make me do it, nor is there anything anyone can do to prevent it. I choose with my actions.

You can give me tools, but the choice to use them, or not, is up to me. There is nothing I will go through that someone else hasn't gone through before me and overcome. That is why capturing the stories about hope, the "how-to" for hopeful mindsets, is key to this work. We must learn from others.

I think back to my own attempt, and the loss of my dad, which is really what this lesson is all about. Internalized failure. We internalize failure so often, without ever knowing it.

Addiction distracted me enough to manage life, albeit only temporarily and superficially. This unaddressed sense of failure, this deep sense of hopelessness of purpose, is what ultimately led to my suicide attempt. I literally believed I was put on this planet to make my dad happy. And I failed. I thought that meant I was a complete and total failure.

I know now that it was not my job to save my dad. Instead, my purpose was to love him and be a daughter. *I was not a failure; I failed at saving my dad.* The difference is profound.

Dr. Guy Winch, a world-renowned psychologist and Ted Talk speaker, provided a lesson for Hopeful Minds to teach kids about failure. Failing at something doesn't mean you are a failure; rather, it means that something in your *process* has failed. By deconstructing the process, you can make adjustments and do better the next time.

We ask our kids this in Hopeful Minds: When you do badly on a test or assignment, what does it say about you?

The answer might surprise you. It says absolutely nothing about you. The reason you fail at things has very little to do with who you are or how smart you are. Instead, the reason you fail has to do with how you go about the process (studying and working).

When you fail or do poorly, it isn't because there's something wrong with you. It is because there's something wrong with your perception of the problem or your method of preparing. In order to improve your methods, you first must overcome a tricky reality: feeling disappointed, discouraged, annoyed, or even helpless.

Although these feelings can be quite strong, they're also incorrect. Some of us might need to put in more effort or do things differently than others, but every one of us can perform well. We just need to figure out how.

To do better, we first need to conquer the negative feelings that send us incorrect messages and confiscate our hope.

The best way for our upstairs brain to create hope is to feel more in control of the situation, and we can help our upstairs brain feel more in control by taking action. But what action should we take?

Consider a student failing a test, and think of the reasons this could happen:

- Students didn't give themselves enough time to study or prepare. Perhaps they didn't keep up with homework and reading, which left too much to learn in the remaining time.
- Students gave themselves enough time but became distracted and didn't use the time well.
- The studying method wasn't effective (e.g., students read the chapter in their math book but didn't do practice problems).
- Students didn't understand the material well enough.
- Students became nervous and had trouble concentrating during the exam or project.

Once they've identified the reasons the students may have done poorly, you can help the student figure out what to do differently. Our Hopeful Minds curriculum goes through this in detail.

If we feel that we are failures, we don't have hope because hope is learning how to detach from failure. Viewing failure from a place of objectivity allows us to do better next time. And it stops us from beating ourselves up.

This book isn't perfect. I can't even imagine the mistakes you've noticed already, though, hopefully, you are letting me know. Our curriculum isn't perfect. The key is to learn and get better. Research. Improve. Fail Forward.

I am a living lab, and it is no surprise that my work on happiness was put to the side so I could focus solely on hope. I had way more to learn, many more emotions to process, things to be healed. I'm so grateful that I've been off medications for over 5 years, do therapy only as needed, my relationships with men are way better, and I'm healing my limiting beliefs on finances.

So really, overall, I'm doing pretty well. My failures aren't crippling me. I'm recovering faster. I'm failing smarter.

And no, I didn't fail at saving my dad. I couldn't save him. And as tragic as his death was to me, I turned that pain and despair at losing him into my calling.

The failure made me work toward ending the global epidemic of suicide. It inspired me to work on myself. So while I couldn't teach my dad how to keep himself alive, I've learned from that process and am using it to try to keep myself, and others, not just alive, but hopeful and happy.

Are there places you have failed in your life? Are you embracing the failures? Learning from them? Encouraging your kids to do the same? Your colleagues?

Better yet, are you *enjoying* the challenges that your failures represent? That is when you know you are a master. I'm still working on that one!

Think like a queen. A queen is not afraid to fail.
Failure is another stepping stone to greatness.

—Oprah Winfrey

RUMINATING ON NEGATIVITY

But keeping on working and hoping still:
For in spite of the grumblers who stand about,
somehow, it seems, all things work out.
—Edgar Guest

What is the rumination of negative thoughts? "I'm a failure. I'm a failure. I'm a failure. I'm a failure. I'm a failure. I'm a failure."

That's rumination.

It can be anything: "My friend doesn't like me." "I ate too much." "I said something stupid," repeatedly in the brain.

Nobody ever tells us that we do that. I wish someone had told me when I was 7 that I was doing it, and ***what a waste of time it is***. I've spent so much time listening to things over and over that made me feel horrible, and I did it to myself.

Now, when a bad show comes up on the TV, I leave the room. I never used to do that. I just let my brain absorb the badness, until I became aware of what I was doing and learned how to avoid it.

Ruminating negativity is holding on to feelings of failure or disappointment. We go over them in our heads, which interferes with our hope tools. Letting the problem persist without intervention sets us up for trouble.

Imagine the following scenario: You're at work, the day seems to be going smoothly, and you're looking forward to a relaxing evening at home. Then, with 15 minutes left, your boss approaches you and informs you that you have done badly on a project. You apologize and try to explain what happened, but all your boss tells you is that you need to get your act together.

Everyone must deal with situations like this from time to time, and it would put most people in a bad mood. You have two options to deal with the situation.

Option #1:

- Spend 15 minutes problem-solving what needs to change and what you will tell your boss the next day, then put the issue aside and enjoy the rest of your evening.
- Let the problem eat away at you, leading you to contemplate how unfair the world can be, how mean your boss is, how much you hate your job, and that you are going to quit. Then taking it home to your spouse and family, being irritable, complaining, and spreading negative emotions around.

Option #2: Ruminating on negative thoughts about the past.

Continuously thinking about the various aspects of situations that are upsetting can easily make the situation worse. Some people never develop a solution to the problem.

Think about what you do. When something upsets you, do you mull on it and keep going over the problem? Ruminating on the problem will keep that negativity alive and, if you keep the negativity alive for days, chances are you'll remain upset for days. How do you respond to distressing situations?

Ruminating on negativity is also connected to many different forms of self-sabotage. For example, if you continue to think about something upsetting a friend did, it's going to take longer to forgive that friend and get back to enjoying time spent with them. If you hold a grudge, you may lose that friendship completely.

It is important to get to the bottom of the problem and come up with an effective solution based on what you can and can't control. Healthy behaviors to distract from the mindset are important. There are many healthy activities that can be used to distract from ruminating on negativity. The best one to use is the one that works for you.

One by one, I've worked hard to replace unhealthy behaviors with healthy ones. When my mind starts ruminating on negativity, I grab a book, go for a hike in nature, take a hot bath, listen to an inspiring YouTube video, get a massage, meditate, head to the gym for a run, do some jumping jacks, watch a good movie, or look at funny videos. These are all used not as an escape from the problem, but to break the repetitive negative patterns of the brain.

There is a subtle difference between escaping behaviors and redirecting behaviors. I believe it is important. If, for instance, you play video games to de-stress, do you feel better or worse after? Are the behaviors negatively impacting your life, relationships, work, or health? Are you drinking a glass of wine because you enjoy it, or to not deal with your issues? Only you know the behaviors that help you shift your mindset out of rumination, and into a better place.

When I was little and had nightmares, my grandma would come in, sit by the side of my bed, and tell me to change the channel. I didn't realize this was ruminating, and that I did it during the day too. I just knew I was having nightmares while I slept.

She told me that if I didn't like the movie playing while I slept, I could watch something else. It worked wonders for me when I was sleeping. The good news is we can do it during the day, as well.

When we teach kids hope, we ask them: If you were watching a bad TV show, would you keep watching it? Not one kid raises his or her hand and says 'Yes.' It is the same process with negative mindsets— if you don't like your thoughts, change the channel.

If you have done the SMART Goal, changed the channel, and tried the other techniques, but you are still ruminating, try sensory engagement. Touch something. Smell something. Taste something. As we mentioned before, you can't be in your mind and the present moment at the same time.

When was the last time you can think of when you were ruminating? How did you get out of it? Was it a healthy behavior? How might you incorporate some of these strategies?

Hope begins in the dark, the stubborn hope that if you just show up and try to do the right thing, the dawn will come. You wait and watch and work: you don't give up.
—Anne Lamott

HOPELESSNESS

*The secret is not to give up hope. It's very hard not to
because if you're really doing something worthwhile
I think you will be pushed to the brink of hopelessness
before you come through the other side.*

—George Lucas

As I mentioned, hopelessness is both a feeling of helplessness and negative emotions. You can feel hopeless about one specific thing (i.e. finances), or about everything in your life. It can slowly creep up on you or hit you all at once, or it can creep in, one thing after another, until you are overwhelmed by it all.

One thing is crystal clear to me; hopelessness kills.

We can be hopeless about so many things—finances, relationships, families, careers, health, the environment, and more. Literally, anything at all can feel hopeless.

I've got to be frank. I've managed suicidal ideations my entire life. If you can take a moment, let that sink in: I've thought about wanting to die since I was in my teens. It actually pops up regularly in my brain as a solution to my problem(s).

Whose brain does that?! Unfortunately, mine.

I rarely talk about it, as I find it annoying, and I believe what we focus on expands. I also don't want to freak people out, as I don't ever plan to do it and am still shocked I made a serious attempt in my 20s. Still, it is my reality, and I've got to be proactive and manage it.

Fortunately, my skills around how to create, maintain, and grow hope keep me focused on the right things. It is all a battle in my mind, and it is a battle I always plan to win.

As stated at the beginning, hopelessness is both a negative feeling and helplessness. If I take no action and stay in a negative mindset, my hopelessness continues. I do everything I can, each and every day, to proactively manage my hope.

I heal my emotions as opposed to running from them. I exercise first and foremost. I just celebrated 17 years of sobriety.

I pay attention to my feelings of hopelessness around many subjects, and work this program diligently to proactively tackle them, so they don't get so out of control.

I also reach out to my network for hope, and communicate honestly where I am. If I feel so hopeless I might self-harm I tell my family and either stay with them for support or go to a treatment center with 24-hour care.

I don't 'threaten suicide' to control or manipulate others into doing something, as that does not heal me. I do the inner work to understand why I don't feel strong enough to solve my own challenges. And I get myself to a place where there's support so that I can, and do.

By threatening suicide, we give our power away and become victims. Yet we really don't know how to tell other people how poorly we feel, and we don't feel capable of solving them, so it makes sense to communicate it this way. When we get others to do our bidding because of these feelings, we just prolong our necessity to deal with the underlying issue.

I couldn't learn to stay alive until I solved the root of the problems that were putting me into hopeless states to begin with. I could lean on people for support, yet I needed to stop getting myself into hopeless situations in the first place, understand how to handle my own emotions, get into a positive place, and create SMART goals so that I could take inspired actions.

If we really want to feel better, we've got to step up to the plate. There is nothing someone, somewhere, hasn't overcome in life. We need to learn from them, not have someone give us a temporary fix. I mean, think about it, how good does that even feel?

To those who experience suicidal ideations, or ever consider it as a solution to a temporary problem, I encourage you to consider a new approach. I feel you, and the statistics, suggest my likelihood of dying by suicide is high, yet every choice I make, every day, writes my story. I aim to beat the odds. I hope you do, too.

Let your hopes, not your hurts, shape your future.
—Robert H. Schuller

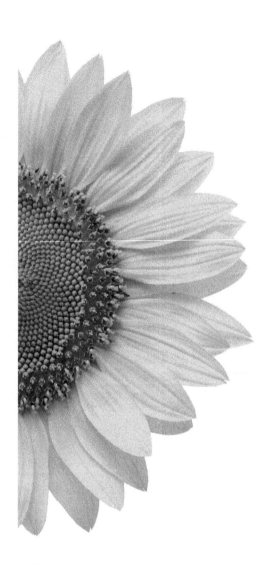

STRATEGIES FOR HOPELESSNESS

When you do nothing, you feel overwhelmed and powerless.
But when you get involved, you feel the sense of hope
and accomplishment that comes from knowing
you are working to make things better.
—Pauline R. Kezer

HOPE NETWORK AND CONNECTIONS

If you are broken, you do not have to stay broken.
— Selena Gomez

oneliness is a global epidemic and, as we mentioned in the original research, hopelessness is a predictor of loneliness and suicide. That is why putting together a Hope Network is so important on your journey to hope. Humans are social beings that need other people, and we can't always tackle hopelessness alone.

Having people to turn to in times of need is crucial. Hope connections offer the unconditional love we need to grow and encourage us to make healthy choices in life. It is important that we take a deep look at our relationships to make sure we are surrounding ourselves with people who add to our hopeful mindset.

When I quit drinking, I had to get serious about my network for hope; everyone I knew at the time drank. I met people in recovery and relied on my therapist and group therapy to keep myself supported, and I made sure that I had a healthy place to turn to in times of need.

When I went through my divorce, I reached out to my family because I was literally devastated to end my marriage. It triggered every feeling of abandonment, failure, and loss of connection, even though it was something I needed to do for my health. I felt shame, and hopelessness about all of the great challenges ahead of me. I was alone and completely overwhelmed.

For the first time ever, I got real with my family about my suicidal ideations, in the spirit of sharing my intense grief. I didn't know what to do. I knew I didn't want to die, yet I didn't know what to do. I was in so much pain.

In sharing my grief and feelings of hopelessness, my big brother Arnold suggested I move close to him and his family, a pretty brilliant move on his part. I was living in the middle of nowhere in Maryland, near no one I knew. His suggestion literally saved my life, as it gave me the strength to look not at all of the hopeless areas of my life (finances, love, company, nonprofit, etc.) but instead to take micro-steps to get my mental health back on track.

I stopped worrying about all of my problems and focused on micro solutions. I focused on fixing my mind, healing from the loss of my dad. I stopped worrying about everyone else for once and focused first on myself.

Slowly but surely, I built my life back up. During that hard time, my mom and my brothers were my Hope Network, my angels. I could not have done it without them and my very close friends from high school who also loved me—no matter what.

Sometimes we have different networks for different goals and challenges in life. I now have an advisory board of experts for my program on hope and can call any of them, anytime, and they will lend an ear to my latest challenge. I have connections for my company who patiently listen to my goals, offer suggestions if they have them, and encourage me to do what is best for myself.

These advisors don't judge me, shame me, ridicule me, or belittle me. My Hope Networks listen and provide support when I feel I have no options left. That alone helps tremendously.

I've got a network of sober friends who keep my ego in check. While I don't have a compulsion to drink or smoke, I am compulsive and impulsive by nature. My ego is strong, yet having these individuals also working a program helps me stay on top of all the various ways I run from pain if I am not careful. They call me out, in a gentle and loving and nonjudgmental way. My amazing Hope Network keeps me grounded in The Now and supported on my journey.

I am also the Hope Network of others. They know they can call me any time to discuss anything, and that I'll try to be a sounding board. I'll listen and encourage healthy behaviors and habits. If it is one of my friends in sobriety and they relapse, I won't cheer them on and encourage them to drink or put themselves in danger. Instead, I'll listen with empathy and offer resources they may consider if they want to get support. What they do is up to them.

I'll share what we know works. I'll set healthy boundaries, continue taking care of myself, and be a good friend. It's just as important to have a Hope Network of your own as it is to be in someone else's Hope Network. We benefit so much from giving time and energy to others.

I encourage you to think both about your own network and those you support. If you can't think of anyone you can support, you can always contact someone like Big Brothers, Big Sisters, a retirement community, or a suicide hotline. There are many people who would love your encouragement in their time of need.

The ocean is wild and over your head
And the boat beneath you is sinking
Don't need room for your bags
Hope is all that you have
So say the Lord's prayer twice,
hold your babies tight
Surely someone will reach out a hand
And show you a safe place to land

Be the hand of a hopeful stranger
A little scared but you're strong enough
Be the light in the dark of this danger
'Til the sun comes up
—Sara Bareilles and John Legend
Excerpt from song; A Safe Place to Land

HOPE SUPPORTER

All kids need is a little help, a little hope,
and somebody who believes in them.
—Magic Johnson

I t is critical that we have at least one person to talk to in a
time of need or crisis—someone we absolutely trust, who has
our best interests at heart, and who we can go to with any
issue, knowing they will simply listen. That is a Hope Supporter.
Hopeful Minds makes sure every child has identified at least one
person as a Hope Supporter. When they can't identify someone,
that is a red flag to the teacher; the teacher becomes that person
of support.

In the middle of a crisis is not the time to think of a Hope
Supporter. We need to have support ready. A Hope Supporter can
be a peer and a great resource for promoting hope. The use of peer
support has helped change the culture of mental health from illness
and disability to health and ability (Mead et al., 2001).

A Hope Supporter is someone who knows and appreciates you, sees your strengths, and helps you keep a hopeful mind. A Hope Supporter is imperative to our hope. It's always important to *ask for help*.

Take a minute to think through some different categories of support:

- Friends on whom you can count
- Family members with whom you feel comfortable sharing your feelings
- A relative (e.g., aunt, uncle, cousin, grandparent) with whom you can talk
- Faculty and staff (e.g., teacher, counselor, coach) you can go to for support
- Colleague/Co-worker
- Teammate or Classmate
- Someone you might be able to count on even though you are not always close
- Therapist or doctor

Sometimes these people can't help us, or our crisis is immediate. There are now many free, global resources to contact when we are in emotional distress. Our Hopeful Minds program includes a personal resource survey, adapted by Dave Opalewski, one of our Hopeful Minds advisors.

The Crisis Text Line is a global not-for-profit organization providing free confidential crisis intervention via text message. The organization's services are available 24 hours a day, every day, throughout the US, UK, and Canada, and can be reached by texting HOME to 741741, 85258, or 686868, respectively.

We list other resources on our website at www.ifred.org. Searching online for a "crisis hotline" in your country often leads to a local resource. It is important to keep these numbers handy and programmed in your phone in case you ever feel yourself needing support unexpectedly. I've listed other mental health resources at the end of the book.

WONDER, AWE, AND FAITH

Hope arouses, as nothing else can arouse,
a passion for the possible.
—William Sloan Coffin

F aith is a touchy subject for many, so we add wonder and awe as
science is supportive of their value. One could create an entire
book on this subject alone. And I would be remiss not to say
that spirituality quite certainly saved my life.

I didn't get there in a straight line and have my own beliefs
about what spirituality means to me, yet I would not be alive without a belief in something greater than myself helping me on my
journey. The connection to that, paired with wonder and awe, has
kept me alive when my network, positive feelings, and inspired
action were just not working for me.

It is rare, but it happens. Because of my brain's thought that
nobody understands me, I feel negative emotions, and I can't think

of one Inspired Action to take. That is when I rely even more heavily on wonder, awe, and faith.

Research supports that Religion and Spirituality are associated with many positive mental health outcomes, including hope (Koenig, 2012). Harold Koenig did an extensive study on all research to date and, while the research is quite compelling, I will note that one size does not fit all, and we all need to make our own decisions about what this means to us. Hope is a human right, and if what you believe is working for your positive feelings and inspired action, that is all I care about.

I wasn't always a believer in God. For many years, I rebelled against religion because my dad died by suicide and some religions proclaim that he is in "Hell" as a result. There is nothing evolved, or positive, about that statement, so I railed against religion. Yet my anger and rejection were just as unevolved, and not coming from the upstairs brain.

I found the anger didn't serve me, either, as it put me 'against' something and was driven by negative emotions. This is just as harmful, so, instead, I let the anger inform me and put the universe to my own tests. In the end, what I rejected was the fear, pain, and isolation that religion could summon if taken to extremes.

It was always my belief that religion caused pain. Yet this isn't really the case; humans cause the pain. Unevolved humans, living in their reptilian brain, are driven by fear, anger, and pain. When I started seeking the positives of religion, learning from the beautiful awe-inspiring insights of the various theologies around the world. I learned a lot, and it made me a better person. I focused on what resonated with me leaving the rest behind.

I settled on a sort of deep spirituality, driven by curiosity and my continual asking of the universe and receiving answers in unexpected and delightful ways. I can't tell you how many times answers came to challenges I'd sent out to the universe—something greater than myself—that were too synchronistic to explain away by mere coincidence.

I don't believe in an angry or spiteful God. I believe that is a God people created from their trauma or misinterpretation, based on their ego and need to control and repress. Religions don't create wars; people do in the name of religions. When we work from our most evolved part of the brain, violence has no place. Aggression is us acting from our reptilian brain.

I believe in an evolved God—a hopeful, loving, and forgiving God, one of divine kindness that connects us all. We humans punish ourselves enough. The God I feel is the one that lifted me out of bed, seeking only to unconditionally love and heal a very broken young woman.

Everyone needs to choose what they feel is best for their own positive emotional state and inspired mindset. In my personal experience, sometimes all the hope tools in the world do nothing for me. I do all the practices, talk to my Hope Network, yet feel so alone that the only thing that can hold me is my spirituality and sense of faith and awe and wonder in the world. Handing it over to the universe, believing something greater than myself is supporting my journey, is a great gift I give to myself.

Just a few weeks ago, feeling frustrated about my finances, I wanted to know why my dad wasn't here to help. I needed to change my mindset. I took my dog Yoda, and out we went, hiking in nature. I spent the first 30 minutes bawling my eyes out, wishing for my dad, asking why I had to be left all alone in this world to fight for myself when my dad was the finance guy, not me. There was a visceral feeling of his absence, a pain I could not shift.

It is amazing that even after 30 years, the feelings can be so raw, but they are what they are. Instead of running from them, I let them flow through me. I asked the Universe (or God, or the Divine, or whatever word you choose to use) why I was left alone and what I was supposed to do.

On this particular day, I looked up and on the side of a hill a few hundred feet away I saw a lone, brown stallion grazing. I cocked my head a bit, in awe, and started making my way up to it, bringing Yoda by my side so he wouldn't chase him away.

I have an affinity for animals, especially horses. I've seen many wild herds on my hikes and am grateful each time, as I learn from them. I see them on about 10% of my hikes, 99% of the time in herds.

The stallion looked at me and continued grazing. I sat about 50 feet away in absolute wonder. I noticed scars on this wild horse's body, yet was inspired by his ease, grace, power, and sureness. I basked in his beautiful energy.

I was reminded of the grace, beauty, and extraordinary power that resides in me. And I realized, perhaps fully for the first time, that I am actually incredibly skilled at finances. I remembered how I managed budgets exceptionally well at American Express, always on time and within guidelines.

I thought about how I'd paid off my debts, each and every one of them, even though some financial institutions had sold them so many times I had to spend hours tracking them down. I thought about how I raised over a million dollars for a program that is used around the world, in different cultures, and is going to live on regardless of my involvement. I thought about how I created a product line from scratch and sold over 9 million of its items.

I finally understood that my limiting belief of 'needing my dad' for finances didn't serve me. Not only did it not serve me; it wasn't true. I needed to let it go. So on that day, with that wild horse on that hill, I did.

I can in no way say that this was a gift from God or the Universe. I don't know how those thoughts came into my mind, or how the horse appeared. I just know that when I needed it, an inspiration from an animal appeared and stopped me. I became present, and received a beautiful message. I was taken out of my negative emotions into extreme presence through sight and sound. I was in wonder and awe.

I know many who have been harmed by religion. I don't believe in this kind of religion, and I don't believe religion is here to traumatize. And I believe all have access to hope. So if religion has traumatized you, then I think it is important you find connection, wonder, awe, and sacredness in other ways. As I believe those are all critical to hope, and hope does not exclude.

I have no interest in convincing you what to believe, just know that if you want to have hope, you must have inspired feelings and positive action. I share only what has worked for me. Take what works for you and leave the rest.

I have called out thousands of times for signs, synchronicities, and solutions to daunting challenges where I do not see hope, and have always been answered. Maybe not in my timing, or in my way, yet I've always been answered. Call it whatever serves you, do whatever works for you.

The most important thing for me is, you always find your way to hope.

Our program, Hopeful Minds, teaches kids about awe, sacredness, and finding something greater than ourselves in times of distress. We don't talk about a specific religion, but we do share the message that when things get too big to handle, giving it over to something greater may help. We let the students define for themselves what that is to them, and use nature, religion, animals, or the beautiful expansive sky as examples.

There are now courses on awe and wonder, and research supporting the power of the positive feeling to our mental health. Buried in our phones or sitting behind our computers, we often fail to take in the magic of the world. It is a lens we are losing. Part of our work is our intention to bring that back.

Taking the time to connect with something sacred, something bigger than ourselves, is so important for our hope muscle. We must hold on to that image, despite what others are thinking, saying, or doing, because sacred things help us see the world outside of ourselves.

I talked about my experience of trying to overdose in my early 20s. I can't help but believe something greater than myself saved me, and that it helped define my mission and get me on track to share my unique perspective with the world.

Maybe I'm wrong, and I have no attachment either way, but I often wonder why this is a force that feels so much greater than me. And why, every time I try to walk away, something unexplainable happens. Who knows? Just because science cannot yet prove it does not mean it isn't real. We must have an open mind and continue to learn.

This works for me, it keeps me alive, and life is better for me with wonder, awe, and spirituality. Studies suggest that, with some exceptions, spirituality is beneficial for hope, happiness, and many other life outcomes. Choose what feels right, and best, for you.

When was the last time you truly felt awe and wonder? How can you add more wonder and awe into your life? How can you inspire others to do the same?

GIVING THE TOOLS OF HOPE

A leader is a dealer in hope.
—Napoleon Bonaparte

Melinda Gates, in an interview with Oprah, talked about one of her most crushing experiences to date. She explains about a time when a new mom in India tried to hand Melinda her baby, saying, "I can't have any more children. I don't have any hope for these two children. I have no hope. I can hardly feed these kids. My only hope is if you take these two boys home with you."

This hit a nerve with me, as I felt the hopelessness of both women in that scenario. The feeling of Melinda not being able to do anything for that woman, and the hopelessness of the woman not being able to care for her child. It was a tragic exchange.

It also highlights the core of our work: You can't *give* someone hope. We can write messages of hope, we can give people tools, we can teach people what makes us *hopeful,* we can share how others have done it, we can empathize when they don't have hope, we can get them to safety… but we can't give them hope.

Hope is an inside job.

It reminds me of the proverb, "Give a man a fish and he will eat for a day. Teach a man how to fish and it will feed him for a life-time." (Of course, the gender needs to be updated to reflect current times, but you get the meaning.)

We can solve people's problems in the short term, but that doesn't do them much good in the long run. What is more helpful is to teach them how to solve problems and create solutions. That is what we aim to do with our curriculum.

If you watch the BBC documentary "Teens on the Edge" in Northern Ireland, you will see Mandy teaching Hopeful Minds to a classroom in Northern Ireland. What I find astounding about this is that just the previous year, her daughter Ellie died by suicide, a tragedy of epic proportions. Yet what a gift to this class, to have Mandy there teaching these skills for hope. What a beautiful way to keep Ellie's legacy alive through the art of giving these tools. This is how we give hope.

Creating these tools for myself gives meaning and purpose to the loss of my dad. It gives my personal pain meaning and allows me to create something positive from it. And while I can't give someone hope, or eradicate their hopelessness, I can share what we know from the research and what I have found from personal experience. What anyone does with that knowledge is up to them.

We know that giving and gratitude are important for hope and instill positive feelings in both parties, which is why we also built it into Hopeful Minds. In the program, we have kids write encour-aging messages to incoming students to wish them well on their hope journey. They plant sunflowers for hope to experience nature or create and erect a sunflower statue to engage their creative juices. On that statue in front of the garden, they put our website, so that other people can also learn the tools of hope—for free. It is a way to share the message and work together. Gardening and creating art are powerful for mental health.

The incoming spring students then read the messages of hope and harvest the sunflowers, saving the seeds to plant the next spring. It showcases the importance of the cycle of hope, and the continuation of giving. It is a gift that does not end.

The importance of giving and gratitude also helped us create Hopeful Cities (www.hopefulcities.org) and Hopeful Mindsets (www.hopefulmindsets.com). Hopeful Cities, an iFred.org project, was created to take Hopeful Minds to the next level – to a city. It was developed as a marketing plan in action that operationalizes hope as it creates awareness about its importance.

Hopeful Cities provides cities around the world with a collection of free and some paid resources that they can use to implement hope throughout their communities and aims to equip the "how-to" of hope wherever it is needed: in the workplace, community, schools, and at home. It is based on other program like Cities for Kindness, and Compassionate Cities, yet focuses on Hope as a skill. We ask that cities around the world sign up to participate, and celebrate the First Monday in May as the official 'Day for Hope' and celebrate it globally, as we do for Compassion, Peace, Happiness, and more.

Hopeful Mindsets was created based on my understanding of hope and framework for 'how' I teach hope, and the work of leading experts on Hope, Mindset, Mental Health, Stress, Positive Psychology, Business, Communications, and more. Each of the Hopeful Mindsets courses is designed to use expert interviews, hope science, and the testimonials of those with lived experience to address the unique challenges that we face in the workplace, in college, in recovery, and beyond.

The initial Hopeful Mindsets course, Hopeful Mindsets on the College Campus, teaches college students and educators how to proactively manage stress, channel emotions in a positive way, take inspired actions through goal-setting, create strong and nourishing networks, eliminate challenges, and effectively create personal change for the better. The ten-lesson course teaches the science of happiness, mental wellness, connection, and hope. It is my hope to continue creating Hopeful Mindsets courses for all different people.

How do you incorporate giving into your life? How does it feel when you give to others? Do you solve problems or teach skills? How might you incorporate the skills of hope into your own work? How might you teach someone hope?

We must die with Hope intact.
—Fred Rogers

MY VISION FOR HOPE

It is hope that gives life meaning. And hope is based on the prospect of being able one day to turn the actual world into a possible one that looks better.
—Francois Jacob

My belief is that hope is a human right. If every person knew how to have a hopeful mindset, we would live in such a different world.

Sustainable development goals would be so much easier to meet, as each person would individually be trained to positively create solutions with Inspired Action from daunting challenges. The very nature of 'how' we teach hope is that we teach 'how' to set a vision for the future, and feel good and take action, and that is really what the Sustainable Development Goals are all about. Yet how can we expect to reach these goals if we don't teach people how to feel good and actually achieve goals?

There is really no challenge that others have not gone through and risen above. While circumstances may not be exactly the same, there are similarities and lessons that can be applied. It is what leads me to my great vision for hope.

The Hopeful Mindset Training platform is an online learning platform where we take each of these lessons and apply them to specific challenges and/or populations. We then interview experts in the field and people who have successfully overcome those challenges. We compile snippets for each lesson, including their specific insights on the "how-to" of hope in order to provide free lessons for all. As always, we teach through the art of story—for peers, by peers.

At this time, we only have one Hopeful Mindsets Training course: Hopeful Mindsets college campuses. It is my hope that we can continue to expand to other populations, including rising from poverty, rebuilding from natural disasters, thriving after having been sex trafficked, overcoming addiction, getting out of homelessness, leaving a gang, becoming a caregiver, and more. While I know these are extraordinarily challenging scenarios, they are all populations that predict high levels of anxiety, depression, and hopelessness. And, be assured, there are people who have succeeded and risen above them.

I want to find these stories, share their methods, and increase levels of hope in these specific populations. As we know, hope is a protective factor for anxiety and depression.

Just as Melinda Gates can't tell the woman in India how to help raise her child out of poverty, I can't provide tips to stop ruminating or alleviate anxiety after a natural disaster. I can't share the feelings one would feel firsthand or suggest how to set SMART goals to rise out of it. And really, if I did, who would listen to me?

The best person to share the message? Someone who has risen from that situation. These are the people we want teaching the "how-to" for specific Hopeful Mindsets.

I want to find those women in India who have successfully cared for their families, even when they felt no hope at times, and get their stories on our platform. I want to have a tool, so that Melinda Gates doesn't have to experience feelings of hopelessness herself. I want Melinda and that woman to come out of that conversation feeling positive and inspired.

And I'd like sunflower gardens, artwork, and photography brought to life around the world to showcase an image of hope that directs people to that learning platform. I'd like to drive the message that hope is teachable and measurable. And I'd like to get people gardening, creating art, sharing, and learning.

I'd like the curriculum modified, improved, and built upon, and I would like to create curriculums for every age level. I'd like it all compiled in a place that is free and accessible to all, in every language, so that people anywhere can see for themselves the power of hope.

I'd like communities to be measured on their levels of hope and companies rewarded for instilling hope. I'd love for each and every person to feel a sense of hope and know where to turn when they don't have any, so that they never give up.

I'd like a Global Night for Hope, where artists and celebrities share their messages of hope with the world. Where they play songs of hope with the world. I'd like it live, broadcast by all the networks, and recorded in Virtual Reality, so people can experience it in the future. I envision a historic event for hope, one that sets hope on fire.

I'd like us celebrating an International Day for Hope, together. Sharing science, stories, and strategies for hope. Learning about the latest work in the field, and what is working and not working.

I'd love murals for hope around the world, artwork, photo exhibits, and more. I'd love to see cause marketing campaigns, improved research, and stories shared. I'd like to continue building together our knowledge and wisdom and making sure each and every person has access to the 'how to' of hope while having an organization that is thriving and evolving.

I really do see a world someday where suicide is only in the history books—a world where people don't feel the need to give up because they know society will support and embrace them in times of need—a world where it is easier and cheaper to get therapy than it is to get a gun.

It's a big, bold vision for hope, and one that will take time. Today, I'm glad to write *The Biggest Little Book About Hope* and add what I can to the knowledge base by sharing what has worked for me, what I have learned through the incredible researchers who have studied hope, and what we have learned from the kids who have studied Hopeful Minds. Because I can't do it all by myself, or in a day, I need all of you.

And as we now know, we can often become hopeless if our goals are too big. We need to chunk them down. My goal was to finish the book, and get it released. To share what I know with the world. I wrote down the goal and had a team to support me in the process and keep me accountable.

I honestly believe that there is nothing more important than to teach people how to have hope. Hope has saved my life and continues to do so to this day. I am committed to hope, and plan to practice it for a lifetime.

I want to see my nieces and nephews grow up. I want to be around for my brothers as they reach new milestones. I want to travel and explore with my adventurous, amazing, inspiring mom. I want to find my life partner, from a healthy and healed place, not from one of need. And I absolutely, 100%, refuse to be another suicide statistic.

If you are reading this, right now, you are helping me keep that dream alive. And for that, I thank you. And I encourage you to join the movement in any way you feel inspired. As hope is a journey we all must take together.

What oxygen is to the lungs, such is hope to the meaning of life.
—Emil Brunner

FROM HOPE TO HAPPINESS

Happiness is when what you think, what you say, and what you do are in harmony.
—Mahatma Gandhi

I put my company to the side for the last few years for a few reasons. Probably the most important one is that I wasn't in the most hopeful place, and still had some healing to do around my dad. Reno, Nevada was a great place to do that.

I also needed to secure my knowledge and understanding of hope in order to live it, breathe it, and certainly to teach it. Getting involved in the work in Northern Ireland, presenting at conferences, doing focus groups with kids, and studying in different cultures has been key to my own understanding. Writing this book has given me insights I didn't even realize I needed.

Furthermore, I got super-excited about what we were learning about hope, and one human can only do so much. I value humility, yet I cannot tell you how amazed I am at the fact that we showed a decrease in anxiety and depression in youth with our program in Northern Ireland. Even if I don't do anything else around hope, if this book touches another, or inspires more programs, I am incredibly grateful.

While my company sponsored a lot of the initial work on hope and, while I love the work I do on hope, I aim for Happiness in life as well. I do believe it is my ultimate mission, as it allows me to do what I am really good at (launch products and talk about moods in everyday language) and raise money for mental health through Cause Marketing, which also eradicates stigma. We really need funding for mental health.

It also allows me to engage with my research-driven and logical mind, launching products that are evidence-informed, while collaborating with the most brilliant researchers in the world. Experimental psychology, logic, statistics, and research are the fields that are second nature to me.

My big bold dream extends beyond hope… to happiness. It is to get my sensory engagement line at The Mood Factory (www.themoodfactory.com) in retail stores, create an app that helps us manage mood states using biological measures, self-reports, and data, to relaunch the 21 Days to Happiness course (and others), to teach about the 90-second stress response, and generally improve moods and presence globally. I'd like to run a consumer products company for moods, taking moods mainstream, raising money for mental health charities around the world, and create an experiential retail environment encouraging others to do the same.

I believe I am better at launching products with a purpose, talking to the press, and eradicating stigma through this work, than trying to raise money to teach hope; people do not seem to want to pay for prevention. We doubled colored light bulb sales at Lowe's, in an SKU x SKU comparison, using unique merchandising, cause marketing, celebrity engagement, and press. We sold over 9 million products. We got the world talking about mental health. We did "social impact" before it became mainstream.

While 1 in 4 people may have mental health conditions at any given time, 4 in 4 have moods, and we need to be intentional about managing them. We have way more power than we think. We have the ability to choose, each moment, what we do to impact how we feel. We've got to do way more work, each and every one of us.

So, there you have it. I've said it 'out loud'. I will keep practicing my own hope and happiness daily and see where it takes me. I will make my dad's wish for my happiness come true and maintain my hopeful state along the way.

I will use my Hopeful Mindset to work to make it happen, and when and if I need to give up on the company, I will do so and know when the time is right. My hopeful and healthy mindset is first and foremost.

And I'll keep reaching out to retailers and see who wants to engage with me on sensory products. I've come to understand we cannot just feel good, we can train ourselves to feel good using the sense of smell. I've got a full scent line based on this research, and we can raise a ton of money for mental health (a lot more than through light bulbs).

I stopped doing light bulbs based on research that blue light keeps us awake. It isn't as simple as that, and not 100% accurate, yet it is the basic reason I stopped. I didn't want to confuse consumers and wanted an evidence-informed approach for my company.

I still have big dreams for the company. I am ready to move forward again, to grow it based on lessons learned from the past. Perhaps I am meant to, perhaps I am meant to focus on hope for now. I am okay with either. I'm not attached to the outcome.

Every day, I wake up and aim to feel good and take Inspired Action. I set SMART goals and know they may change, and I practice the art of the pivot and am open to when I regoal. I catch my rumination and worry, and shift them. I stay present.

I am grateful. I keep my network for hope strong, and I am a hope supporter for others. I surrender to where I am. I give it over to the Universe. I find wonder and awe. I experience and release my negative emotions and get help when necessary.

I choose healthy habits, and don't beat myself up if I fail. It isn't that I am a failure, it is that my process failed. So I deconstruct the process. And no matter what life brings, I find my way back to hope. And happiness.

I'm grateful to say these strategies, for me, work. I've been off medications and self-managed for five years. I've been sober for 17 years. Just this year I passed the milestone of reaching 50, making it past the amount of time my dad was here on this earth. I'm beating the odds.

I'm open to going back on meds if I need them, and have a therapist for if and when I need extra help. I get sleep. I manage the suicidal ideations by always asking myself 'What am I hopeless about,' and I make sure to focus on solving that problem.

This may or may not work for you. All I can do is share what I know, and what we have learned with our work. I take hopelessness, and hope, very seriously and aim to give others tools I didn't have and that took me a long time, and a lot of money and pain to learn.

Thank you again, for reading my story, listening to my journey, and allowing me to share my own personal vision.

May you also, always, find your way to hope. And if you so desire, be so bold to even find happiness.

> *No matter where you are on your journey,*
> *that's exactly where you need to be.*
> *The next road is always ahead.*
> —Oprah Winfrey

AFTER HOPE

Once You Choose Hope, Anything's Possible.
—Christopher Reeve

know, almost done. I swore I was going to keep it short, but I really can't make this up. Remember the Franchise Board, where this all began? I forgot to finish the story.

It has been several months since that initial call. Since then, I've been writing this book, adding parts when I have time in between my consulting, The Mood Factory, and iFred / Hopeful Minds work, plus the holidays. It's been a busy time.

And clearly, I didn't go home and do anything drastic. I stayed and had a wonderful holiday with my mom and family. I made it through the period of hopelessness with flying colors. I took it one day at a time, one action at a time, and life has been pretty amazing.

I ended up going back and forth with the board many, many times. For months. Lots of communications on my end, little on theirs. Frozen assets twice. Lots of stress; lots of stress management, using all of these tools.

Getting documents from my accountant, talking to different specialists, going around in circles. Faxing my taxes. They said it didn't match with their records, yet they couldn't show me what they had. It went around and around, and I practiced my hope tools.

I remained positive. I did my best not to get annoyed and anxious, though I'm pretty sure on the last few calls I was not 100% smiley. I kept up my healthy eating habits, got my exercise, and kept my network for hope strong.

I said thank you when I talked to them and made micro-goals my purpose.

All in all, Positive Emotions, Inspired Action, with a vision to overcome this challenge in life.

And I kid you not. The very day I finished this manuscript, I got a call from the Franchise Board. They found the problem. It was identity theft and fraud. Somehow, some person got all my information and filed taxes on my Social Security number in California, with a few other businesses, so they could get deductions. What a mess.

It's all resolved. The very day I finished my work on hope.

I wasn't even going to finish the story. I had forgotten all about it. I wish I were kidding. I literally called my mom crying (joy tears).

These are the kinds of things, quite regularly, that keep my faith strong. That keeps me on my journey. That reminds me I am on the right path.

So, a special shout-out to Marcus, who finally resolved this for me. It helped me get over my last bit of fear that this was a dumb book, that it was silly to put it out into the world, that it was TMI (too much information), and that I didn't need to share my story. Coincidence or not, it sealed this book's fate.

So, to add to that list of gratitudes, I'm thankful for the IRS. That's it. All done. The end.

SHINE FOR HOPE

Just when I think it is over, there is more. That is the nature of research and a scientific mind; you test a hypothesis, get feedback, improve, adopt, and relaunch. So it should be no surprise that since I started writing this book, we've made tons of advances in our work.

One of the most important things we've done is work very hard to make hope easier to understand and more organized. In doing so, we created "The Five Keys for Hope," along with a mnemonic SHINE that you will start to see in our work moving forward:

Stress Skills
Happiness Habits
Inspired Actions
Nourishing Networks
Eliminate Challenges

SHINE basically combines everything we spoke about in this book, yet creates a more easily digestible format and structure for people to remember and understand. We've updated our curriculums, worksheets, 10 Day Challenge, 30 Day Challenge, Hopeful Mindsets on the College Campus program, Workplace Campaign, and more. I thought about doing it for the book, yet there is something really beautiful about seeing where the work started and where it is going.

Most people don't start projects because they want perfection right away. If I had thought that way for hope, I never would have started. My 10 lesson curriculum is in many ways an embarrassment, yet as with any hypothesis, you start somewhere and test, test, and test again.

The key is to be clear you don't know it all, and are learning. Many people have asked, "who are you to teach hope?" I'm not anyone, I'm just the one that got tired of hearing about suicides, feeling suicidal, and not knowing what to do about it. I got sick of the way we treated mental health, and so, instead of complaining, I got to work.

I didn't get millions in funding for research, so I bootstrapped it all. And I kept at it, I kept improving, and I kept working on my own mental health and understanding of hopelessness. Figuring out how to teach hope, and keep it free globally for young kids, has touched on an even deeper hopelessness within me that has forced me to continue practicing the Five Keys to Hope necessary for me to make it through.

And here we are today: not perfect, but always improving. We don't have the power to save every person's life, as we cannot do the work for anyone. However, we can give people the tools and, if a person continues to practice Stress Skills, Happiness Habits, Inspired Actions, Nourishing Networks, and Eliminating Challenges, they are on their way.

We all need to SHINE for hope, especially during these challenging times when there are so many things to be hopeless about. We must all collectively and actively practice these skills, and teach others to do the same.

May our work, these tools, and your critical and important feedback continue to improve our knowledge of hope, hopefulness as a society, and collective work towards a better future for us all.

WAYS TO SPREAD THE MESSAGE

If you are so inspired, I'd love for you to join us in helping spread the message of hope. We need you. Seriously. There are tons of ways you can support hope:

- Bring *Hopeful Minds* to your schools and teach a child. www.hopefulminds.org
- Bring *Hopeful Minds* to your local community center, Girl or Boy Scout Troop, Big Brothers & Big Sisters group, Boys & Girls Clubs, mentoring program, church, or more. It is free, and the lesson plans are all online.
- Ask your local University to partner with us on research for our program, or Hopeful Mindsets, or sponsor a student in taking it. www.hopefulmindsets.com
- Take the Global Hope Challenge with family, friends, or colleagues. https://globalhopechallenge.com/
- Plant a *Gardens for Hope* sunflower garden in your community and put up a sign directing people to Hopeful Minds. If you can't plant a garden, consider putting up an art installation or sculpture. www.gardensforhope.org
- Ask your company to sponsor hope in the workplace, increase communications on mental health, and invite Kathryn to speak on hope.
- Sponsor a *Hopeful Workplace* campaign. https://hopefulcities.org/hope-in-the-workplace/
- Donate to hope via iFred, a 501c3 that runs this program. www.ifred.org. It's tax-deductible.
- Tell a friend about hope.

- Share *The Biggest Little Book About Hope* with your friends, family, colleagues, or ask your company to give it to employees. Have a seminar on the "how-to" of hope at the workplace.
- Ask a celebrity to do a PSA on hope. Hope needs a serious rebrand, and celebrities are well-equipped to get the message out. It is a muscle you can build; it is measurable; it is teachable. And it is free for all. Who knew?! https://hopefulcities.org/create-public-service-announcement/
- Practice your hope skills. Daily. Hourly. Every minute. Every second.
- Have your organization partner with us to create *Hopeful Mindsets* training for targeted populations. https://hopefulmindsets.com/
- Create a Hope app with us (would be amazing!!)
- Create or sponsor a Hope bot, so we can practice our hope skills regularly for free.
- Do a Cause Marketing campaign for hope, supporting hope on the front of your product while raising money for iFred (or ask a company to do one).
- Run a *Sunflowers for Hope* photography contest, and feature at your local museum. You would be amazed at the images people create from sunflowers.
- Sponsor a *Hope Challenge for Teens,* where they create a program on teaching hope to their peers, using our framework.

The opportunities are as unlimited as your imagination, so feel free to get inspired and in touch! Help spread our message for hope and get the tools in the hands of all who need them. Feel free to reach out at hope@ifred.org, anytime.

I'll do my best to get back to you, but we don't have staff now, so patience is a virtue. And thank you, thank you, THANK YOU, for helping us spread this work.

ADDITIONAL RESOURCES

This book is for information only, a personal perspective to share what I know about hope. It should not be used as a substitute for medical advice, counseling, or other health-related services. If you are in crisis in the US, call 800-273-TALK (8255) or text HOME to the Crisis Chat line at 741741.

Check out our website at www.ifred.org for additional resources and information. We have an online community for support. Our Hopeful Minds curriculum booklet is free, and available on our website. There are so many great resources out there, doing incredible work for mental health. Here are a few:

- American Academy of Child & Adolescent Psychiatry: http://www.aacap.org/
- American Foundation for Suicide Prevention (AFSP): https://afsp.org/
- American Psychiatric Association: https://www.psychiatry.org/
- American Society of Clinical Psychopharmacology: www.ascpp.org
- Anxiety and Depression Association of America (ADAA): https://adaa.org/
- Big Brothers, Big Sisters: https://www.bbbs.org/
- Black Lives Matter: https://blacklivesmatter.com/
- Born This Way Foundation: https://bornthisway.foundation/

- Children's Mental Health Network: https://www.cmhnetwork
  .org/
- Cities Rise: http://cities-rise.org/
- The Clay Center for Young, Healthy Minds: https://
  www.mghclaycenter.org/
- The Depression and Bipolar Support Alliance: https://
  www.dbsalliance.org/
- Dignity and Power Now: http://dignityandpowernow.org/
- Erica's Lighthouse: https://www.erikaslighthouse.org/
- Fundamental SDG: https://www.fundamentalsdg.org/
- Global Coalition on Youth Mental Health: https://
  ymentalhealth.org/
- Grief Recovery: http://www.griefrecovery.ws
- Healthy Place: http://www.healthyplace.com/
- Hopeful Minds: https://hopefulminds.org/curriculum/
- Hopeful Minds Parent Guide: https://hopefulminds.org/
  curriculum/
- International Association for Suicide Prevention (IASP):
  http://www.iasp.info/resources/Crisis_Centres
- International Foundation for Research and Education on
  Depression: https://www.ifred.org
- Inspire, iFred's Anxiety and Depression Support Community:
  https://www.inspire.com/groups/ifred-anxiety-and-depression/
- The Kennedy Forum: https://www.thekennedyforum.org/
- The Lovell Foundation: https://lovellfoundation.org/
- "The Mask You Live In" Documentary: http://
  therepresentationproject.org/film/the-maskyou-live-in-film/
- Matthew Ornstein Foundation: https://www.mornstein.org/
- Mental Health America: https://www.mhanational.org/

- Movement for Global Mental Health: http://globalmentalhealth.org/
- National Alliance on Mental Illness (NAMI): https://www.nami.org/Home
- National Council for Behavioral Health: https://www.thenationalcouncil.org/
- National Institute of Mental Health: http://www.nimh.nih.gov/index.shtml
- One Mind: https://onemind.org/
- Peg's Foundation: https://pegsfoundation.org/
- Pretty Girl Passion Society: https://www.prettygirlpassionsociety.com/
- PsychCentral: http://psychcentral.com/
- The Scattergood Foundation: https://www.scattergoodfoundation.org/
- "Screenagers" Documentary: https://www.screenagersmovie.com/
- Steinberg Institute: https://steinberginstitute.org/
- Substance Abuse and Mental Health Services Administration: http://www.samhsa.gov
- Treatment Advocacy Center: https://www.treatmentadvocacycenter.org/
- The Trevor Project: https://www.thetrevorproject.org/
- Voices around the World: https://voicesaround.com/
- Welcoming Schools: https://www.welcomingschools.org/
- Well Being Trust: https://wellbeingtrust.org/
- Women's Brain Project: http://www.womensbrainproject.com/
- World Dignity Project: http://theworlddignityproject.org/

- World Health Organization: http://www.who.int/en/
- Youth Mental Health First Aid: https://www.mentalhealth firstaid.org/populationfocused-modules/youth/
- Zimbabwe Friendship Bench: https://www.friendship benchzimbabwe.org/
- Thrive Global: https://thriveglobal.com/

IN CELEBRATION

This book is a celebration of my mom and two brothers. They are first in my network for hope, have kept me hopeful in the most trying of times, and have always been there for me no matter what. They have brought me laughter, joy, adventure, hope, happiness, and kids (my inspiring nieces Sarah, Maura, and Clara, and nephew Charles). They are the anchors of my life, and I celebrate them in my heart each and every day.

IN HONOR

This book is in honor of my dad, who died by suicide when I was only 19. I'm releasing the book on February 20, 2020, the 30th anniversary of his passing. Strange, as in many ways it feels like yesterday.

This book is a summary of the work I have done since then to understand his disease, the cause of suicide (hopelessness), and figure out why I could not save him, try as I may.

The memory of that day lives in every cell of my body. I miss you, Dad. I want you to know that you have not died in vain.

I have used your loss to build a legacy of hope and happiness, bringing the brilliance you shared with me in business to make it accessible and sustainable for all. You would be so proud of and love the kids around the world I am meeting who are learning about the power of hope. I am certain they would have loved you.

This book is also in honor of me. For fighting my own hopeless demons every day, even when the statistics are against me. I have most of the risk factors of dying by suicide. It is in honor of me not giving up and instead choosing, every day, to stick around even when the going gets tough.

My ambitious goals and inner voice don't always give me the easy road. Sometimes it means I walk a solitary path. My lived experience of anxiety, depression, PTSD, ADHD, suicidal ideations, addictions, a previous attempt, and more, have collectively made my journey more challenging and stacked the odds against me. So, I honor myself in this book, and the continuous choice of hope and, even so boldly, happiness, *no matter what.*

This book is also in honor of all who struggle with anxiety, depression, addiction, PTSD, ADHD, schizophrenia, bipolar disorder, or other conditions that cause one to feel marginalized, discriminated against, alone, unsupported, afraid, and often hopeless. I want you to know that I see you. I feel you.

I honor your struggles, the way you do your very best despite the pain inside you. Your courage never ceases to amaze me: the challenges you overcome, and the obstacles that you find your way around. You have no idea how much you inspire me.

There are many outside influences telling you that your lived experience is your crutch, or it isn't real. We now know better. There is a biology and behavior interplay, and we are learning more every day.

I believe, once you accept your challenges and channel them for good, your diagnosis will become your superpower—your gift with which you can change the world for the better. This book is for you, and I am cheering for you along the way.

This book is in honor of those who have lost loved ones to suicide. The pain is like watching someone drown and not being able to save them. It never goes away, and that is OK.

I honor your strength for carrying on, after you have seen a brother, uncle, cousin, father, sister, mother, child, friend, colleague, or other lose their struggle to hopelessness. It is so very, very painful.

While we can't save others, we can save ourselves. You can make your own life meaningful again. I wish for you healing and that you find purpose in your pain.

May you someday KNOW, deep within yourself, that it wasn't your fault. May my own lived experience, insight, and knowledge help make that a bit clearer for you. May you finally believe you *are* enough, that you *did* enough, that it was not your fault. This book is for your strength and recovery. Know that I wish you peace and healing in your journey.

This book is a tribute to all who have died by suicide. I write this book in honor of all of you. Each and every one of you.

As a society, we failed you. Our fear of the unknown adds to the stigma, and we know so little about mental health. We isolate those who are different, as opposed to loving and seeking first to understand. I'm sorry we didn't have enough resources to support you and that you did not feel any sense of hope at the end.

Know now, for certain, that millions are stepping up to invest in mental health and work tirelessly to ensure that we eradicate suicide and hopelessness once and for all. We are doing it for all of you. We love you, and we miss you.

And lastly, this book is for anyone who has ever felt hopeless, about anything at all. The world can be a hard place, and there are many challenges each and every one of us faces. Yet it is also a beautiful, magical, incredible place of awe and wonder.

May this book support you in finding your own way, in all ways, and always, to hope.

IN GRATITUDE

I am grateful to so many people. I've left the specifics for the end of the book. I want to give some general thoughts of gratitude here.

This book would not be possible without those who have stepped up to be father-like figures to me, filling that ever-present void in my life. My dad was a great loss to me, as he was larger than life. You can imagine the hole that was left behind. In time, instead of missing him so much, I started asking the universe to give me dads who could help me on my journey. Myron, Paul, Barry, Jim, Larry, and Tom, my two brothers, Arnold and Fred, and so many more, including my ever-amazing mom- Thank you.

I'd also like to thank the friends who have cheered me on and stayed with me through the ups and downs of my recovery to self. My community in Oak Park and friends at the University of Iowa, you got me through the toughest period of my life. Thank you.

And to those who have supported iFred, planting sunflower gardens, putting up signs, teaching hope, engaging with celebrities, doing social media, and creating videos. And then, of course, those who supported The Mood Factory: packing boxes, shipping press kits, visiting stores, helping with research. Thank you; it has all made this work possible.

I'd like to thank the celebrities who have spoken of their struggles of hope and supported me with my Cause Marketing for Mood-lites. Those at the *Teen Choice Awards,* who engaged with me when I was up against Ugg Boots and the Apple Dog and said how much you loved the charity for its mental health component, I thank you. Your early encouragement of iFred let me know I was on the right path, even 15 years ago when stigma was strong and social entrepreneurs rare. I wouldn't have been brave enough to do it without you. So, thank you.

And as boring as gratitude can be to read, do me a favor and read the section at the end anyway. It matters. These people I am thanking are *Champions of Hope,* so send them love for moving the needle and changing the way the world sees people. They are bold adventurers, taking a stand for human rights. They are true heroes.

I am forever indebted to you as well, for reading this book and sharing this message. Thank you for listening to my story and learning about this work. I pass on to you the torch of hope, to carry this work forward. Shine it brightly, whenever and wherever possible.

MY INFINITE GRATITUDE

Feeling gratitude and not expressing it
is like wrapping a present and not giving it.
—William Arthur Ward

I used to breeze over this part of books, as I found them irrelevant. Now I know better. Gratitude is one very powerful ingredient of hope. So now that I know how critical gratitude is to hope, I relish every 'thank you' in books, read the names to myself, and send that energy their way. I bask in the glory of gratitude; it feels amazing.

My gratitude begins with my family. First, a general thank you to all of them. I know that talking about my dad, constantly bringing up the loss, is not easy for anyone. And sometimes I wish I didn't feel compelled to, yet again I believe it inspired hope and happiness, and that is a beautiful thing. As it is ultimately about my dad's quest, how he inspired my work, and how I want him remembered.

I first need to honor my mom, who has energetically joined me on this journey of hope and happiness by being on my board, editing my materials, planting sunflowers, packing Mood-lite boxes (which supported this work), working trade shows, licking envelopes, listening to my woes, investing in me, and encouraging me on my path. Her willingness to put my healing first and fulfill my passion in this world is so inspiring. She has been there for me every step of the way, and I could not be more grateful.

Fred, my brother for whom I named iFred, helped me through many depressive episodes and often cheered me up when I was struggling as a kid. Whether it was blasting Bruce Springsteen's 'No Surrender' or playing 'Bridge Over Troubled Water' by Simon and Garfunkel, he was and is a safe place for me to land. And, of course, I am grateful for his incredible wife, Katherine, and my so fun and adventurous nieces Maura and Clara, and the entire Ryan family, who bring me unbridled love and joy and adventure. You're all amazing and I love you so much.

To Arnold, my oldest brother, who has bailed me out of trouble more than once. When I was feeling horrific after my divorce, he came and moved me to Ann Arbor to be near family. When I couldn't afford to pay rent, he moved me out of my house and turned his 'garage project' into 'his sister's house' project. And not only did he do it; he did it without complaining, judging, or shaming. He pretty much saved my life by helping me recover, bit by bit, and shared his two kids, Sarah and Charles, whom I love and adore, with me. Arnold is a lifesaver, and I'm so happy that he found Marina, who inspires me in so many ways as she boldly pursues her dreams in nursing.

My gratitude includes my mom's husband Larry, a consistent, steady, and stable force and father figure to me. Someone who willingly brought me into his own family. I'm especially grateful for

Darla, who has supported and encouraged my work each step of the way. Even before I have finished the book, she is requesting copies for her friends. She is extraordinarily kind, and never ceases to amaze me with her shining example of hope.

And to my extended family- aunts, late uncle, and cousins- I love you all so much. Even if we rarely talk, I know you are always there, and I am always here. I am so grateful to have you in my life, and you have all supported me so much on this journey.

I wouldn't be here without my friend Kirsten and her family, who have taken me (and my many dogs) in on more than one occasion, always with open arms and a loving home. They follow me on my adventures, cheering me on the whole way. Anton, her enthusiastic husband, is like a brother to me, and Sophie and Jack, two of the brightest and coolest kids I know, lifted my spirits with exciting trips to Great America and game nights at home. This family, and Barb and Hans, and Ty and Jen, have kept me rooted and grounded, always opening up their homes to me when I venture a little too far out of my comfort zone. It is so nice to still have a place to call home in my hometown of Oak Park, IL.

Thank you to my strong, bold, beautiful, inspiring female friends: Cammie, Madeleine, Cherie, Kim, Gina, Aileen, Steffani, Renee, Jen, Christy, Jennifer, Amanda, Deana, Neeta, Ritu, Natalie, Mindy, Kathy, Sandy, Kirsten, Kristy, Stacie, Colleen and the entire Maroney family, Lindsey, Catherine, Lizzy, Michelle, Frankie, Lynn, and so many, many more. No matter how far away we live or how long it has been since we last talked, you are always there for me. My world is better because of you.

I thank those who were willing to step in and become surrogate dads to me for my business and work. To the late Paul Carter, the late Peter Ross, Barry Litwin, Dr. Myron Belfer, Tom Dean, and the newly adopted Jim Foorman. Having you all in my life is a gift that has allowed me to continue solving challenges as they arise. Your steadfast kindness has given me strength. Knowing you cared about my dad, hearing the stories, keeping his legacy alive, helps me. Seeing me through my business challenges, believing in my vision. I cannot thank you enough. The most significant hole in my life has been filled by your love, dedication, support, encouragement, and guidance.

Myron, you will never understand the impact you have had on both my work and the global work of hope. Your guidance, encouragement, kindness, generosity, and wisdom have helped me through some of the hardest times. Your ability to see beyond where my addictions and trauma brought me, to where I brought myself through my work and dedication, has given me faith in humanity. Every piece of wisdom you have given me has served me well. You are the definition of an angel.

To the late Paul Carter, who, beyond being a dad, helped keep Walmart alive for me with the Saturday morning meetings when my dad could no longer take me. The place where I first saw Nancy Brinker speak about The Susan G. Komen Foundation, breast cancer, and her vision for the future. I had imagined that same trajectory for mental health, knowing the power of Walmart and retail. I took in every encounter, listened closely, and thought about how it might apply to mental health.

To the entire Carter family, including June, Stephanie, Sam, Steve, and Michelle. It is no surprise to me that after I sent my book to Amazon, I went out to the mail and got a card June sent me with a pic of my dad and thank you card he had sent to Paul years ago, congratulating Paul on an achievement. June, your love, kindness, warm heart, and notes from the past have meant the world to me. Your actions keep my dad's memory alive. Stephanie, your strength and modeling of hope and faith. Steve, your sound business advice and compassion. Michelle, your warm energy and sense of humor. Sam, your willingness to support me even though you don't know me as well as the rest do. And all the grand and great-grandkids, I love you all so much.

Paul was such a wonderful man, and through his generous gift of time, informed so much of this work. He was a great role model in my life, another beacon of hope helping me rise out of addiction, showing me you didn't need to drink to fit in. His love of family, commitment to his faith, and the way he handled his emotions all made an impact on me. I'll never forget the story about him on the call with a supplier. He didn't raise his voice, he stood on top of his desk, and expressed to the supplier, 'I'm so frustrated I'm standing on my desk'. He didn't threaten, punish, or demand, or act against the person in anger; he shared his feelings and got on his desk. He committed to solving the challenge in a way that worked for all. What a great lesson on hope.

Thank you to the late Sam Walton, who also taught me business didn't need to revolve around alcohol and that it is important to stand up for what you believe in. He taught me the power of a smile, and the importance of connecting with people. The 10-foot rule and the concept 'Lose your smile, lose your customer' is everything you need to know about the power of hope and happiness; it even impacts retail, and Sam had such foresight in the power of kindness and connection. And the late Helen, a strong woman who taught me the importance of community and family. I feel so blessed to have been a part of the very early years; they warmed my heart and influenced my journey greatly. Helen and Sam's values, commitment to others, kindness, humility, and warmth stay in my heart.

That my dad was such good friends with Sam and Bud, that my dad saw the vision of Walmart in the very early stages, really highlighted to me what a great loss it was to the world to have him leave so early. I cannot even begin to imagine what my dad may have created if he'd had the tools he needed to stick around. I feel lucky to have spent time with the Walton family in those very early years.

To Lynne Walton, who purchased my initial light bulbs off my website. That one purchase gave me faith in my vision. That maybe I could make my dad proud, and maybe I was onto something. Since people who knew him, who did great things in life, cared about me and paid for my products. It gave me a little bit of hope to take that next step.

To Jim Walton, who met me at Arvest Bank long ago to talk about my dad, sharing stories. To Rob, who answered my messages and encouraged my mission in life. Rob taught me the art of surrender and the belief that I must never give up, though he may not even be aware of it. Rob, let me recount getting stuck in a storm with you on a Saturday morning float trip, when you built me a fire, a memory that keeps my dad's legacy alive.

While I have not connected personally to Alice probably since a young child, I want to thank her for so much. Her love for animals, nature, and art still inspire me and is so much a part of hope. Crystal Bridges Museum in Bentonville is one of the most extraordinary art museums in the world, and I've seen a lot. Alice's contributions to the world improve Hopeful Mindsets in so many ways by investing in creativity, something so often undervalued in academia, yet key to success in life. Alice is a real visionary.

I am grateful for my amazing schools, Mann, Hawthorne, and OPRF, and the incredible friends and supporters who got me through challenging times. To my friends at the University of Iowa, Winona, Green Bay, Australia, Africa, and St. Thomas: Thank you. I'm not sure how I made it through any of my schooling considering my life at the time. It was only possible because of you. The fact that I graduated college in 4½ years, even with all the transfers and my active addictions, was a miracle. If 'lived experience' were a Ph.D., I would have gotten it from Harvard.

Thank you to Christine, my first official sponsor after 14 years of sobriety. Your beauty, encouragement, strength, and laughter have taken me through next-level sobriety and healing. It has been a fun few years, and I have learned so much from you. And thank you to all those in my sober community, as your stories and depth give me strength in recovery and remind me I am not alone. Recovery is not possible without each and every one of you.

Thanks to all my therapists, clinicians, doctors, and psychiatrists, especially Jennifer and Arlene. Thank you for guiding me back to hope. Gently. Compassionately. Encouragingly. You'll be so glad to know I'm doing awesome. I wouldn't be here without your love and support. Thank you to Maureen Muldoon, who taught me how to have fun with spirituality, the importance of consistency, and the magic of miracles. Thank you to Esther, who taught me the art of alignment, and that I didn't have to wait on another's actions to feel a certain way. Thank you to Mark, Felix, Robin, and all the other spiritual leaders and teachers who have inspired my journey back to myself and God.

Thank you to Michael Singer, for teaching such a powerful lesson on business about the elusive and ineffective 'chase'. Thank you for giving me permission to stop running after it, and start just being. I was really tired. Thank you for taking the time to connect live, allow me to share my story, and give me further insight into your work so it may inform mine. You are a gift to me and this world.

And to all of the men in my life who have helped me on my healing journey. Thank you for your love, forgiveness, kindness, and care. Thank you for helping me become a better woman. Thank you for letting me heal from the loss of my dad and, in general, my fear of men. Thank you for your unconditional love, most especially John, who taught me the meaning of the word and how to love myself. Thank you to the entire White family, who took me in as one of their own, I love you all so much.

Thanks Rohan, Mike, Steve, Brandon, Brad, Adam, Michael, Asa, David, Ashraf, Brian, Mark, Miles, and E, for encouraging the mission and journey, and for being the evolved men I so love to see in this world.

To my investors, advisors, and supporters of The Mood Factory. My program on hope would not be alive without my company's initial success. Scott Mandell, Beth Pacenka, Kirsten Straughan, Dave Lampson, Dr. Nadim Shaath, Dr. Rachel Herz, Dr. Ehud Baron, Dr. Elizabeth Lombardo, Leatrice Eiseman, Dr. Myron Belfer, Sprint, Dave Meltzer, Kimberly Green-Kerr, Jeff Klinefelter, Alan and Aaron Feit, Jeff Slaboden, Mark Kleinhenz, and so many, many more. Thank you, thank you, thank you. I'm looking forward to Mood 2.0.

To Anna, who sits beside me, continuing to fight for hope and happiness as best she could over these last few years. What a true inspiration. Thank you for your dedication to our vision, and for continuing to take care of yourself and your family, first and foremost. You are a gem, and this book and our last few years' work on hope would not have been possible without you.

Thank you to my iFred Board of Directors, all of whom have listened to my struggles with empathy, encouragement, and a steady hand. Dr. John Grohol, a true innovator in mental health and a leader in the field. Mindy Magrane, who is a strong female leader I so admire. Tom Dean, who brings structure, guidance, and formality to our work. Jim Link, my professor in business school, who taught me how to create new products and gave me that solid, consistent encouragement I so needed. Your teaching has served me well.

Thank you to the Hopeful Minds Advisory Board, who listened and encouraged me to pursue this work, and provided knowledge and support: Dr, John Boyd, Dr. Barbara Van Dahlen, Sophie Straughan, Matthew Jackman, Chantelle Booysen, Dr. Gabby Ivbijaro, Dr. Moitreyee Sinha, Dr. Myron Belfer, Dr. Guy Winch, Nigel Frith, Dr. Delaney Ruston, Dr. Karen Kirby, Dr. Gary Belkin, Dr. Elizabeth Lombardo, Jim Link, Kimberly Blaine, Kristy Stark, Marie Dunne, Dave Opalewski, John Blake, Nancy Tamosaitis, and Susan Minamyer. In loving memory of Anna Unkovich, an author of *Chicken Soup for the Soul in the Classroom* and a strong advocate for children. Also, to the late Paul Carter, who taught me how to keep going, no matter what, and of our need to teach children with kindness, compassion, and love.

To the incredible Northern Ireland team: Karen, Marie, Wendy, Nigel, Paula, Cherie, John, Aoife, Mandy, Katrina, the incredible kids, and so many others. We would not be here without your research. Your dedication to this dream, with expectations of nothing in return, shows the beauty of the human spirit and force of good in the world. May Ellie live on through this work.

To the mental health leaders and advocates who are pioneers in this field, I've been lucky enough to spend time with you and I've learned so much. Thank you for sharing your wisdom, guidance, and support. You have all informed this work so much; Dr. Maurizio Fava, Dr. Shekhar Saxena, Dr. Pamela Collins, Dr. Vikram Patel, Dr. Arthur Kleinman, Dr. John Boyd, Dr. Gabby Ivbijaro, Dr. Antonella Santuccione, Dr. Phil Wang, Dr. Julian Eaton, Dr. Husseini Manji, Dr. Kathleen Pike, Dr. Walter Greenleaf, Dr. Delaney Ruston, Dr. Harry Minas, Dr. Maria Teresa Ferretti, Dr. Daniel Amen, Dr. Randy Phelps, Dr. Paolo Del Vecchio, Dr. Gary Belkin, Dr. Chip Fisher, Dr. Joyce Marter, Dr. Tom Insel, Sir Graham Thornicroft, Dr. Eliot Sorel, Dr. Greg Fricchione, Chris Underhill, Katherine Switz, Karlee Silver, Mary De Silva, Garen, Shari, and Brandon Staglin, Patricio Marquez, Mary Deacon, Arianna Huffington, Drew Holzapfel, Dr. Gino Yu, Miri Polachek, Maya Smith, Audrey Gruss, Cynthia Germanotta, Brooks Kenny, Brad Herbert, Nicole Votruba, Joe Polish, Luis Gallardo, Talinda Bennington, Charlene Sunkel, Elisha London, Reese Butler, and all the other Global Mental Health leaders and icons that I learn from every day. Thank you for honoring my lived experience and letting me participate in this global activism, sharing hope with the world. It has been a great honor to learn from you all.

Thank you to all of the global funders who are now taking mental health seriously. *Grand Challenges Canada, Wellcome Trust, Pivotal Ventures, The Pritzker Group, Joy Ventures,* and more. Your early adoption created the tipping point we needed. Our collective humanity is grateful.

Thank you to John Boyd and Sutter Health, for helping to keep the vision for Hopeful Minds alive and thriving. Your belief in this work, and your commitment to hope, are so appreciated. We would not be here without you.

Thank you to celebrities who have stepped up for mental health—you are changing the conversation by giving people the courage and space necessary to talk about it: Bruce Springsteen, Lionel Richie, Katy Perry, Lady Gaga, Sheryl Crow, Russell Brand, Sting, Chris Martin, Selena Gomez, Oprah, J.K. Rowling, Stephen King, Russell Brand, Brad Pitt, Brook Shields, Brittany Spears, Beyonce, Kendall Jenner, Adele, Ryan Reynolds, Chrissy Teigen, Michelle Williams, Miley Cyrus, Lena Dunham, Dakota Johnson, Demi Lovato, Emma Stone, Gina Rodriguez, Carrie Fisher, Ellen DeGeneres, Jared Padalecki, Dwayne 'The Rock' Johnson, Lili Feinhart, Nicki Minaj, Kesha, Amanda Seyfried, Winona Ryder, Olivia Munn, Ellie Goulding, Sarah Silverman, Zayn Malik, Kristen Bell, Kerry Washington, Gwyneth Paltrow, Halle Berry, Camila Mendes, Princess Diana, Prince Harry, Cara Delevingne, Glenn Close, Drew Barrymore, Zendaya, Eminem, Kristen Stewart, Ben Affleck, Mariah Carey, Carrie Fisher, Bebe Rehxha, Mel Gibson, Demi Lovato, Brian Wilson, Sia, Ted Turner, Catherine Zeta-Jones, Sinead O'Connor, Hayden Panettiere, Adam Levine, Jim Carey, Elton John, Jon Hamm, Angelina Jolie, David Beckham, Brittany Snow, Olivia Munn, Megan Fox, and so many, many more. Thank you. May we someday all gather to lift the world with our collective strategies and stories for hope.

Thank you to Patrick Kennedy for leading the addiction movement and driving powerful legislation to provide support for those in need. You are an icon for change.

Thank you to the *Women's Brain Forum* for creating conversation about women and leading in research and advocacy.

Thank you to Craig Kramer, for leadership in corporate mental health. Thank you to J&J for starting the *Y Mental Health* movement. There is no doubt about it, youths are our future.

Thank you to Dr. Moitreyee Sinha, for encouraging me personally and professionally, as it relates to hope and happiness. Thank you for helping spread hope through *CitiesRISE* and sharing an incredible team that inspires, motivates, and uplifts my mission and work. I love you all so much.

Thank you to the incredible youth voices around the world that inspire me–Lian, Chantelle, Matthew, and so many more. Never have I been so excited for the future of mental health, with all your bold activism. You are rock stars, thanks for shining your bright lights for the generations to come.

Thank you to Kate Kleyman and Charles Spearman at *Guggenheim Partners* for taking inclusion seriously and letting me share my story in the workplace. The ability to speak with folks in finance, a company so closely tied to my dad, on the positive ROI for mental health and my work on hope and happiness meant the world to me. Changing the workplace conversation is key to eradicating stigma; I wonder where my dad would be today had there been such open discussions. I'm grateful you are giving your employees the opportunity to take charge of their own mental health; it will serve them (and you) well.

To all the initial employees, supporters, and encouragers of our work. It has been a bootstrapped ride, which is never easy. I know my demands have been high and I've learned so many lessons along the way. Thank you so much Candice, Mellissa, Melissa, Camine,

John, Alisa, Kristin, Penny, Sarah, Michonne, Beth, and so many more. Thank you for supporting the mission and continuing on your own path in life. You are all so inspiring.

Thank you to all the folks who forgave me when I was deep in my addictions. To those I lied to, cheated on, or disrespected. While I have worked hard to make amends, to those I missed, I'm sorry. To all, your understanding and compassion for my misgivings and faults are appreciated. Forgiveness is a powerful force.

Thanks especially to those who said I couldn't do it, for challenging me to search for answers and truth. It is in those challenges that we find our voice and where we come to understand the necessity of being still, of listening, and sifting out the ego with inspired guidance. Thank you for challenging me to stop running and start listening.

Thanks to my 99 Design winner _Arbëresh_®, and to all those who participated in the cover design process. It was a fun challenge, and a hard decision! I appreciate your creativity.

Thanks to both my _Fiverr_ editors, for helping me sift through all these pages and versions. Caroline Barnhill and your attention to detail at the end. Sunflower_edits for your content and flow suggestions. You were both a tremendous support in the process. Thanks also to those after the fact, including Beth Wood Elliott, I'll always remember you catching that random paragraph of the two oxen and air conditioner. I'm sure I was going somewhere with that story. Classic!

Thank you to Carol Purroy and Taylor Steed, who helped to update, edit, and launch the second edition of _the Biggest Little Book About Hope_.

And thank you to God, as I know you, for helping me move this work forward. Thank you for inspiring these words and for allowing me to serve humanity. May they reach those who need them. I'm grateful I found my way back to you, and to myself. Thank you for guiding me back to hope, and for believing I am worthy of happiness.

And thank you, the reader, for bringing this message to life for me. For taking the time to read the story, learn about hope, and care about humanity. It is only through you that this message gets out to the world.

ABOUT THE AUTHOR

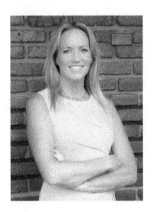

Kathryn Goetzke, MBA, is a social impact entrepreneur, strategic consultant, global mental health advocate, and Chief Mood Officer of The Mood Factory. Kathryn's nonprofit, iFred, created Hopeful Minds™, a free global program featured as an innovation by the World Bank aimed at teaching young kids the "how-to" of hope. She developed Hopeful Cities™ so communities around the world can operationalize hope, and through her consulting developed Hopeful Mindsets™, a method of overcoming challenges through science, stories, and strategies for hope. She is also the host of The Hope Matrix podcast. Kathryn has presented at the United Nations, Harvard, the World Health Organization, been featured on news organizations around the world, and serves on the advisory boards for the

Global Mental Health Movement, Y Mental Health, Women's Brain Project, and FundaMentalSDG, and is a representative of the World Federation for Mental Health at the United Nations Department of Public Information. She grew up in Chicago, Illinois, and currently resides in Reno, Nevada with her dog, Yoda.

BIBLIOGRAPHY

Ajdacic-Gross, V. (2008). Methods of suicide: international suicide patters derived from the WHO mortality database. *World Health Organization, 86*(9). Retrieved February 22, 2020, from 10.2471/ BLT.07.043489

Avey, J. B., Reichard, R. J., Luthans, F., & Mhatre, K. H. (2011). Meta-analysis of the impact of positive psychological capital on employee attitudes, behaviors, and performance. *Human Resource Development Quarterly, 22*(2). Retrieved February 22, 2020, from 10.1002/hrdq.20070

Berendes, D., Keefe, F. J., Somers, T. J., Kothadia, S. M., Porter, L. S., & Cheavens, J. S. (2010). Hope in the Context of Lung Cancer: Relationships of Hope to Symptoms and Psychological Distress. *Journal of Pain and Symptom Management, 40*(2). Retrieved February 23, 2020, from 10.1016/j.jpainsy mman.2010.01.014

Bolland, J. M. (2003). Hopelessness and risk behaviour among adolescents living in high-poverty inner-city neighbourhoods. *Journal of Adolescence, 26*(2). Retrieved February 22, 2020, from 10.1016/s0140-1971(02)00136-7

Borchard, T. (2010, March 4). Why Are So Many Teens Depressed? *Psych Central, World of Psychology.* Retrieved February 22, 2020, from https://psych central.com/blog/why-are-so-many-teens-depressed/

Chester, D. S., DeWall, C. N., Derefinko, K. J., Estus, S., Lynam, D. R., Peters, J. R., & Jiang, Y. (2016). Looking for reward in all the wrong places: dopamine receptor gene polymorphisms indirectly affect aggression through sensation-seeking. *Social Neuroscience, 11*(5). Retrieved February 22, 2020, from 10.1080/1747 0919.2015.1119191

Cotruş, A., Stanciu, C., & Bulborea, A. A. (2012). EQ vs. IQ Which is Most Important in the Success or Failure of a Student? *Procedia - Social and Behavioral Sciences, 46.* Retrieved February 22, 2020, from 10.1016 /j.sbspro.2012.06.411

Courtney, E., Kushwaha, M., & Johnson, J. (2008a). Childhood Emotional Abuse and Risk for Hopelessness and Depressive Symptoms During Adolescence. *WJEA, 8*(3). Retrieved February 23, 2020, from 10.1080/10926790802262572

Curray, L., & Snyder, C. R. (n.d.). Role of Hope in Academic and Sport Achievement. *Journal of Personality and Social Psychol-*

ogy. Retrieved February 14, 2020, from https://web.archive. org/web/20200214004721/https://pdfs.semanticscholar. org/0b86/b27d538384b716c151676b2ead7b786d438d.pdf

Davis-Laack, P. (2019, February 5). The Business Case for Hope. *Forbes*. Retrieved February 22, 2020, from https://web. archive.org/web/20200222211940/https://www.forbes.com/ sites/pauladavislaack/2019/02/05/the-business-case-for-hope-creating-the-future-you-want/

Day, L., Hanson, K., Maltby, J., Proctor, C., & Wood, A. (2010a). Hope uniquely predicts objective academic achievement above intelligence, personality, and previous academic achievement. *Journal of Research in Personality*, *44*(4). Retrieved February 22, 2020, from 10.1016/j. jrp.2010.05.009

Dekhtyar, M., Beasley, C. R., Jason, L. A., & Ferrari, J. R. (2012). Hope as a Predictor of Reincarceration Among Mutual-Help Recovery Residents. *Journal of Offender Rehabilitation*, *51*(7). Retrieved February 22, 2020, from 10.1080/10509674.2012.711806

Duke, N. N., Borowsky, I. W., Pettingell, S. L., & McMorris, B. J. (2011). Examining Youth Hopelessness as an Independent Risk Correlate for Adolescent Delinquency and Violence. *Matern Child Health J*, *15*(1). Retrieved February 22, 2020, from 10.1007/s10995-009-0550-6

Gallagher, M. W. (2017). *The Oxford Handbook of Hope*. Oxford University Press.

Haatainen, K. M., Tanskanen, A., Kylmä, J., Honkalampi, K., Koivumaa-Honkanen, H., Hintikka, J., Antikainen, R., et al. (2003a). Gender differences in the association of adult hopelessness with adverse childhood experiences. *Social Psychiatry and Psychiatric Epidemiology, 38*(1). Retrieved February 22, 2020, from 10.1007/s00127-003-0598-3

Huen, J. M. Y., Ip, B. Y. T., Ho, S. M. Y., & Yip, P. S. F. (2015). Hope and Hopelessness: The Role of Hope in Buffering the Impact of Hopelessness on Suicidal Ideation. *PLoS ONE, 10*(6), e0130073. Retrieved February 22, 2020, from 10.1371/journal.pone.0130073

Jacobsen, D. (2013, May 15). Self-Efficacy, Optimism, Resilience and Hope. Retrieved February 22, 2020, from https://www.workhuman.com/resources/globo force-blog/self-efficacy-optimism-resilience-and-hope

Johnson, T., & Tomren, H. (1999). Helplessness, Hopelessness, and Despair: Identifying the Precursors to Indian Youth Suicide. *American Indian Culture and Research Journal, 23*(3). Retrieved February 22, 2020, from 10.17953/aicr.23.3.vq543623wv51h23t

Joiner Jr., T. E., & Rudd, M. D. (1996). Disentangling The Interrelations Between Hopelessness, Loneliness, And Suicidal Ideation. *Wiley Online Library*. Retrieved February 22, 2020, from https://onlinelibrary.wil ey.com/doi/abs/10.1111/ j.1943-278X.1996.tb00253.x

Keng, S.-L., Smoski, M. J., & Robins, C. J. (2011). Effects of mindfulness on psychological health: A review of empirical studies. *Clinical Psychology Review*, *31*(6). Retrieved February 22, 2020, from 10.1016/ j.cpr.2011.04.006

Killingsworth, M. A., & Gilbert, D. T. (2010). A Wandering Mind Is an Unhappy Mind. *Science*, *330*(6006). Retrieved February 22, 2020, from 10.1126/ science.1192439

Kirby, K., Lyons, A., Mallett, J., Goetzke, K., Dunne, M., Gibbons, W., Ní Chnáimhsí, Á., et al. (n.d.). The Hopeful Minds Programme: A Mixed-method Evaluation of 10 School Curriculum Based, Theoretically Framed, Lessons to Promote Mental Health and Coping Skills in 8–14-year-olds. *Child Care in Practice*, 1–22. Retrieved February 22, 2020, from 10.1080/13575279.2019.1664993

Koenig, H. G. (2012). Religion, Spirituality, and Health: The Research and Clinical Implications. *ISRN Psychiatry*, *2012*. Retrieved February 23, 2020, from 10.5402/ 2012/278730

Lopez, S. J. (2014). *Making Hope Happen*. Simon and Schuster.

May, E. M., Hunter, B. A., Ferrari, J., Noel, N., & Jason, L. A. (2015). Hope and Abstinence Self-Efficacy: Positive Predictors of Negative Affect in Substance Abuse Recovery. *Community Ment Health J, 51*(6). Retrieved February 22, 2020, from 10.1007/s10597-015-9888-y

Mazza, J. J., Catalano, R. F., Abbott, R. D., & Haggerty, K. P. (2011). An Examination of the Validity of Retrospective Measures of Suicide Attempts in Youth. *Journal of Adolescent Health, 49*(5). Retrieved February 22, 2020, from 10.1016/j. jadohealth.2011.04.009

Opalewski, D. (2011). Grief Recovery Inc.: Helping People Grieve and Grow. Retrieved February 23, 2020, from 10.1037 /e550252013-001

Rand, K. L., Martin, A. D., & Shea, A. M. (2011). Hope, but not optimism, predicts academic performance of law students beyond previous academic achievement. *Journal of Research in Personality, 45*(6). Retrieved February 22, 2020, from 10.1016/j.jrp.2011.08.004

Rath, T. (2009). *Strengths-Based Leadership*. Simon and Schuster.

Rath, T., & Conchie, B. (n.d.). Strengths Based Leadership. *Gallup Inc.* Retrieved February 22, 2020, from https:// web. archive.org/web/20200222223922/https://www.gallup.com/ press/176588/strengths-based-leadership.aspx

Roberts, M. (2017, September 20). 1 In 4 Girls 'Shows Signs of Depression.' *BBC News*. Retrieved February 22, 2020, from https://web.archive.org/web/20200222231628/ https://www. bbc.com/news/health-41310350

Roesch, S. C., Duangado, K. M., Vaughn, A. A., Aldridge, A. A., & Villodas, F. (2011). Dispositional hope and the propensity to cope: A daily diary assessment of minority adolescents. *Cultural Diversity and Ethnic Minority Psychology*, *16*(2). Retrieved February 23, 2020, from 10.1037/a0016114

Ruch, D. A., Sheftall, A. H., Schlagbaum, P., Rausch, J., Campo, J. V., & Bridge, J. A. (2019). Trends in Suicide Among Youth Aged 10 to 19 Years in the United States, 1975 to 2016. *JAMA*, *2*(5), e193886. Retrieved February 22, 2020, from 10.1001/jamanetworkopen. 2019.3886

Schiavon, C. C., Marchetti, E., Gurgel, L. G., Busnello, F. M., & Reppold, C. T. (2016). Optimism and Hope in Chronic Disease: A Systematic Review. *Frontiers in Psychology*, *7*. Retrieved February 23, 2020, from 10.3389/fpsyg. 2016.02022

Scioli, A. (2010). *The Power of Hope*. Simon and Schuster.

Sher, L. (2004). Preventing suicide. *International Journal of Medicine*, *97*(10), 677–680. Retrieved February 22, 2020, from 10.1093/qjmed/hch106

Siyahhan, S., Aricak, O. T., & Cayirdag-Acar, N. (2012). The relation between bullying, victimization, and adolescents' level of hopelessness. *Journal of Adolescence, 35*(4). Retrieved February 22, 2020, from 10.1016/j.adolescence.2012.02.011

Stern, S. L., Dhanda, R., & Hazuda, H. P. (2001). Hopelessness Predicts Mortality in Older Mexican and European Americans. *Psychosomatic Medicine, 63*(3). Retrieved February 22, 2020, from 10.1097/00006842-200105000-00003

Tartakovsky, M.S., M. (2011, January 20). Why Ruminating Is Unhealthy and How To Stop. *PsychCentral, World Of Psychology.* Retrieved February 23, 2020, from https:// psychcentral. com/blog/why-ruminating-is-unhealthy-and-how-to-stop/

Thompson, E. A., Mazza, J. J., Herting, J. R., Randell, B. P., & Eggert, L. L. (2005). The Mediating Roles of Anxiety, Depression, and Hopelessness on Adolescent Suicidal Behaviors, *35*(1). Retrieved February 22, 2020, from 10.1521/ suli.35.1.14.59266

Trautmann, S., Rehm, J., & Wittchen, H. (2016). The economic costs of mental disorders. *EMBO Rep, 17*(9). Retrieved February 22, 2020, from 10.15252/embr.201642951

Walton, A. G. (2017, November 8). 7 Ways To Pull Your Wandering Mind Back Into The Present Moment. *Forbes.* Retrieved February 22, 2020, from https://web.archive.org/ web/20200222212656/https://www.forbes.com/sites/alice-gwalton/2017/11/08/7-ways-to-pull-your-wandering-mind-back-into-the-present-moment/

Weir, K. (2013, October). Mission Impossible. *Https://www.apa. org.* Retrieved February 22, 2020, from https://www.apa.org/ monitor/2013/10/miss ion- impossible

Wilson, Dr. D. R. (2018, September 25). Diaphragmatic Breathing And Its Benefits. *Healthline.* Retrieved February 22, 2020, from https://web.archive. org/web/20200222212135/

Winch, G. (2013). *Emotional First Aid.* Penguin.

Zhu, A. Q., Kivork, C., Vu, L., Chivukula, M., Piechniczek-Buczek, J., Qiu, W. Q., & Mwamburi, M. (2017). The association between hope and mortality in homebound elders. *Int J Geriatr Psychiatry, 32*(12). Retrieved February 23, 2020, from 10.1002/gps.4676

Zurbriggen, E. L., Gobin, R. L., & Freyd, J. J. (2019). Childhood Emotional Abuse Predicts Late Adolescent Sexual Aggression Perpetration and Victimization. Retrieved February 23, 2020, from 10.4324/ 9781315874920-10

(2006, November 10). Longitudinal Effects Of Hope On Depression And Anxiety: A Latent Variable Analysis. *Journal of Personality.* Retrieved February 22, 2020, from https://onlinelibrary.wiley.com/doi/abs/10.1111 /j.1467-6494.2006.00432.x

(2012, June). FACT SHEET ON BEHAVIORAL HEALTH CONDITIONS Behavioral Health Disorders – All-Encompassing Condition. *National Association of State Mental Health Program Directors.* Retrieved February 22, 2020, from https://www.nasmhpd.org/ sites/default/files/ Public%20and%20 Private%20 Financing_Fact%20Sheets%20on%20Behavioral%20Health.pdf

(2015). Solution-focused Practice Toolkit | NSPCC Learning. *NSPCC Learning.* Retrieved February 23, 2020, from https://learning.nspcc.org.uk/research-resources/ 2015/solution-focused-practice-toolkit/

(2016, April 12). Investing In Treatment For Depression And Anxiety Leads To Fourfold Return. *World Bank.* Retrieved February 22, 2020, from https://www. worldbank.org/en/news/press-release/2016/04/13/ investing-in-treatment-for-depression-anxiety-leads-to-fourfold-return

(2018a, April 19). Scientists Identify Connection Between Dopamine And Behavior Related To Pain And Fear: New Research Illuminates Crucial Links Between Avoidance Behavior And Key Brain Chemicals. *ScienceDaily.* Retrieved February 23, 2020, from https://www.scienc edaily.com/releases/2018/04/180419131108.htm

(2018b, August 11). How Thoughts Block Us From Being Fully Present. *Psychology Today.* Retrieved February 22, 2020, from https://www.psychologytoday.com/us/ blog/inviting-monkey-tea/201808/how-thoughts-block-us-being-fully-present

(2018c). *Youth Risk Behavior Survey*. Retrieved February 22, 2020, from https://www.cdc.gov/healthyyouth/data/ yrbs/ pdf/trend sreport.pdf

(2019a). The Link Between Alcohol Use And Suicide - Alcohol Rehab Guide. *Alcohol Rehab Guide*. Retrieved February 23, 2020, from https://www.alcoholrehab guide.org/resources/ dual-diagnosis/alcohol-and-suicide/

(2019b). Most U.S. Teens See Anxiety, Depression As Major Problems. *Pew Research Center's Social & Demographic Trends Project*. Retrieved February 22, 2020, from https://www.pew-socialtrends.org/2019/ 02/20/most-u-s-teens-see-anxiety-and-depression-as-a-major-problem-among-their-peers/

(2020). Empathy Definition | What Is Empathy. *Greater Good*. Retrieved from https://greatergood.berk eley.edu/topic/ empa-thy/definition

A free ebook edition is available with the purchase of this book.

To claim your free ebook edition:

1. Visit MorganJamesBOGO.com
2. Sign your name CLEARLY in the space
3. Complete the form and submit a photo of the entire copyright page
4. You or your friend can download the ebook to your preferred device

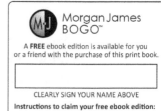

A **FREE** ebook edition is available for you or a friend with the purchase of this print book.

CLEARLY SIGN YOUR NAME ABOVE

Instructions to claim your free ebook edition:
1. Visit MorganJamesBOGO.com
2. Sign your name CLEARLY in the space above
3. Complete the form and submit a photo of this entire page
4. You or your friend can download the ebook to your preferred device

Print & Digital Together Forever.

Snap a photo

Free ebook

Read anywhere

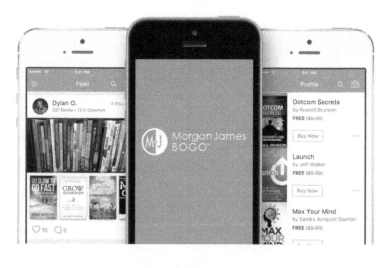

www.ingramcontent.com/pod-product-compliance
Lightning Source LLC
Jackson TN
JSHW081329130125
77033JS00014B/470